Patient-Centered Prescribing

Seeking concordance in practice

Jon Dowell BMed Sci, BM, BS, MRCGP, MD
Senior Clinical Lecturer in General Practice
University of Dundee

Brian Williams BSc, PhD
Senior Lecturer in Behavioural Science
University of Dundee

David Snadden MBChB, MClSc, MD, FRCGP, FRCP (Edin)
Vice Provost Medicine
University of Northern British Columbia
Associate Dean, Northern Medical Program
University of British Columbia

Radcliffe Publishing
Oxford ● New York

Radcliffe Publishing Ltd
18 Marcham Road
Abingdon
Oxon OX14 1AA
United Kingdom

www.radcliffe-oxford.com
Electronic catalogue and worldwide online ordering facility.

British Library Cataloguing in Publication Data

A catalogue record for this book is available from the British Library.

ISBN-13: 978 185775 835 1

Typeset by Advance Typesetting Ltd, Oxford
Printed and bound by TJ International Ltd, Padstow, Cornwall

Contents

Series editors' introduction

The strength of medicine in curing many infectious diseases and some of the chronic diseases has also led to a key weakness. Some believe that medicine has abdicated its caring role and that, in doing so, it has not only alienated the public to some extent, but also failed to uphold its promise to 'do no harm.' One hears many stories of patients who have been technically cured but still feel ill, or who feel ill but for whom no satisfactory diagnosis is possible. In focusing so much attention on the nature of the disease, medicine has neglected the person who suffers the disease. Redressing this twentieth-century phenomenon required a new definition of medicine's role for the twenty-first century. A new clinical method, which was developed during the 1980s and 1990s, has attempted to correct the flaw and to regain the balance between curing and caring. It is called the *patient-centered clinical method* and has been described and illustrated in *Patient-Centered Medicine: Transforming the Clinical Method*, by Stewart *et al.* (2003). In the latter book, conceptual, educational and research issues were elucidated in detail. The patient-centered conceptual framework from that book is used as the structure for each book in the Series introduced here. It consists of six interactive components to be considered in every patient–practitioner interaction.

The first component is to assess the two modes of ill health, namely disease and illness. In addition to assessing the disease process, the clinician explores the patient's illness experience. Specifically, the practitioner considers how the patient feels about being ill, what the patient's ideas are about the illness, what impact the illness is having on the patient's functioning, and what they expect from the clinician.

The second component is an integration of the concepts of disease and illness with an understanding of the whole person. This includes an awareness of the patient's position in the life cycle and the proximal and distal contexts in which they live.

The third component of the method is the mutual task of finding common ground between the patient and the practitioner. This consists of three key areas, namely mutually defining the problem, mutually defining the goals of management/treatment, and mutually exploring the roles to be assumed by the patient and the practitioner.

The fourth component involves using each visit as an opportunity for prevention and health promotion. The fifth component takes into consideration that each encounter with the patient should be used to develop the helping relationship. The trust and respect that evolve in the relationship will have an impact on other components of the method. The sixth component requires that, throughout the process, the practitioner is realistic in terms of time, availability of resources and the role of collaborative teamwork in patient care.

However, there is a gap between the description of the clinical method and its application in practice. The series of books introduced here attempts to bridge that gap. Written by international leaders in their field, the series provides clinical explications of the patient-centered clinical method. Each volume deals with a common and challenging problem faced by practitioners and serves to reinforce and illustrate the patient-centered clinical method.

The book series is international, to date representing Norway, Canada, New Zealand, the USA, England and Scotland. This is a testament to the universality of the values and concepts inherent in the patient-centered clinical method. We feel that an international definition of patient-centered practice is being established and is represented in this book series.

The vigor of any clinical method is proven in the extent to which it is applicable in the clinical setting. It is anticipated that this series will inform further development of the clinical method and move thinking forward in this important aspect of medicine.

Moira Stewart PhD
Judith Belle Brown PhD
Thomas R Freeman MD, CCFP
March 2007

Reference

Stewart M, Brown JB, Weston WW *et al.* (2003) *Patient-Centered Medicine: transforming the clinical method* (2e). Radcliffe Medical Press, Oxford.

About the authors

Jon Dowell BMed Sci, BM, BS, MRCGP, MD is a graduate of the University of Nottingham. He trained in family medicine in Tayside, Scotland, and subsequently joined the academic unit in Dundee. Practicing as a part-time family doctor in Forfar, a small rural town in northern Tayside, he is also a Senior Lecturer in General Practice in the Community Health Sciences Division of Dundee Medical School. Although his prime responsibilities and interests are in education, his early academic career focused on researching the prescribing process and medication use in the primary care setting. It is this primarily qualitative research that has provided the foundation for this book. This work has been published, presented internationally and contributed to the Royal Pharmaceutical Society of Great Britain's 'Compliance to Concordance' initiative (www.concordance.org). His combined interest in education and the consultation has led to extended postgraduate courses for family doctors, specialists and practice-based clinical pharmacists.

Brian Williams BSc, PhD is a graduate of the University of Surrey. His first degree was in economics and sociology, with an emphasis on medicine and healthcare. He was employed for seven years as a researcher within the National Health Service in North Wales, conducting research into patients' experiences of both their illness and service provision. In 1998 he took up the position of Health Services Research Coordinator for Tayside, before being promoted to the position of Senior Lecturer in Behavioural Science within the Department of Epidemiology and Public Health. He has an international reputation in the field of patient satisfaction and patients' evaluations of services, but in more recent years has concentrated on the experience of illness and how these beliefs and experiences relate to behaviors such as adherence. His recent research has examined adherence in the context of schizophrenia, depression, exercise, cystic fibrosis, childhood asthma and the potential benefits of fixed drug combinations (FDCs). He is now the Associate Director of the Social Dimensions of Health Institute (www.sdhi.ac.uk), and is part of an alliance of researchers developing a programme of work around 'self-care' (www.ascr.ac.uk). He is also responsible for behavioral science and health promotion teaching within the Dundee Medical School curriculum.

David Snadden MBChB, MClSc, MD, FRCGP, FRCP (Edin) is a graduate of the University of Dundee. He trained in family medicine in Inverness, Scotland, and practiced as a rural family physician for 10 years in the north of Scotland before taking a Masters Degree in Family Medicine at the University of Western Ontario, Canada. He returned to Scotland to academic practice at the University of Dundee, where he was Senior Lecturer in General Practice and Director of Postgraduate General Practice Education at Tayside Centre for General Practice before becoming acting postgraduate dean. His primary interests are in medical education and family medicine, and his main research activities, including his doctoral thesis, have used qualitative methods to investigate reflective learning mechanisms. He has also researched patient experiences with chronic illness and collaborated with Jon Dowell in the research projects that provided much of the material for this book. He is currently Professor in the Northern Medical Program at the University of Northern British Columbia (UNBC), and affiliate Professor in the Department of Family Practice at the University of British Columbia (UBC) in Canada. He is also Associate Vice President of Medicine at UNBC and Associate Dean of the Northern Medical Program UBC, where his responsibilities are to establish the Northern Medical Program as part of UBC's distribution of medical undergraduate education throughout British Columbia.

Chapter contributor

Nicky Britten MSc, PhD, FRCGP (Hon) is a graduate of the University of Oxford, where she studied mathematics. She then obtained a Master's degree in management science and later a PhD in sociology, both at the University of London. She spent 10 years working on two of the British birth cohort studies before joining the Department of General Practice at what used to be the United Medical and Dental Schools of Guy's and St Thomas' hospitals as a lecturer. She ran their MSc in general practice for many years before joining the newly opened Peninsula Medical School as a professor in 2003. Her research interests include medicines use, patient professional communication, complementary and alternative medicine, and the synthesis of qualitative research. She was a member of the Royal Pharmaceutical Society of Great Britain's working party which produced the document *From Compliance to Concordance: Achieving Shared Goals in Medicine Taking*. At the Peninsula Medical School she is leading a new MSc in integrated healthcare, which offers a framework for studying the potential for the integration of conventional and complementary approaches to healthcare.

Acknowledgements

We thank the Community Health Sciences Division (formerly Tayside Centre for General Practice) at the University of Dundee for providing a supportive environment in which to conduct this research and write this book. In particular we express our thanks to Professor John Bain and Professor Frank Sullivan for their consistent encouragement.

We are of course indebted to the research participants, both patients and physicians, who so generously shared their stories and experiences with us and without whom academic progress in this domain would be impossible.

We would like to thank the series editors for their contributions and challenges, and especially Jana Bajcar for her detailed and helpful suggestions and Andrea Burt for her coordination and attention to detail. Thanks are also due to Professor Pamela R Ferguson, Department of Law, University of Dundee, for advice regarding legal precedent in the UK.

The funding bodies that have supported both the individuals and the studies which have contributed to this work are acknowledged, but we should point out that the ideas and suggestions presented in this book are those of the authors and series editors alone, and no other endorsement is intended or should be inferred.

As everyone who has been through the process of writing a book knows, heartfelt thanks are surely due to those nearest and dearest who have to share the experience, and provide the time and support required by it.

Chapter 1

Introduction

Jon Dowell

The original Greek term for drug – 'Pharmakon' – has three meanings; remedy, poison, and magical charm.

(Montagne, 1988)

This book is about medication use and the prescribing process in the western context. Increasingly, patients want to participate in decisions about their care, and we consider how the 'patient-centered' approach can help this process. In particular, we focus on the difficulties that suboptimal medication use can create and how this issue (often labelled as *non-compliance* or *non-adherence*) can be approached within consultations using techniques based on this philosophy. This problem has vexed clinicians for generations, but the increasing trend towards partnership between patients and clinicians is shifting thinking and offering new approaches. In the UK, the term *concordance* has been coined to exemplify this shift but, to us, this simply represents the maturation of the principles and practice of truly patient-centered care into the therapeutic element of the consultation. Increasingly, it is not seen as sufficient for clinicians to explore patients' perspectives in terms of feelings, ideas, function and expectations and then to direct them as to how to respond – for instance, what medication to take. Sharing decisions about treatment has always been present in the patient-centered clinical method, but the emergence of a literature on how this might be achieved reflects the increasing emphasis placed upon it (Brown *et al.*, 1989). We argue here that there is enormous potential value in understanding this process and building the skills to implement it for two reasons. First, there is ample evidence that medicines are used suboptimally throughout the world, and any means of improving this is worth exploring. Secondly, *non-compliance* commonly undermines the clinical relationship, sometimes including deliberate deceit and making rational advice or decisions impossible. Avoiding or overcoming this trap must be a worthwhile objective.

Just as gathering the biomedical details of a clinical history is based upon an understanding of the potential pathologies involved, it is also valuable to appreciate how patients' beliefs, values and other influences can influence their eventual use of a treatment. In the same way that ideas or fears about a symptom can assist or prevent patients accepting a diagnosis, ideas or fears about medicines will affect their willingness to accept them. Appreciating the range and origins of different beliefs about medicines will enable clinicians to identify symptoms of problems and explore these further, just as they would for physical problems. This book is designed to provide an understanding of the types of problems that underlie ineffective medication use and some tools for opening up this topic with patients. This is not always easy, especially when deceit is involved, and this area is covered in some depth in Chapter 7.

Conceptually it might be helpful at this point to introduce the notion of a spectrum of prescribing. Clearly there are times when patient involvement is not possible, helpful or appropriate to seek, emergency care being the prime example. However, even here patient autonomy is acknowledged through advance directives precluding blood transfusion for Jehovah's Witnesses, for instance. At the other end of the spectrum are choices where the clinical evidence does not allow clear guidance or there may be genuine clinical 'equipoise' (Elwyn *et al.*, 2000). An example of this might be the short-term use of hormone replacement for menopausal symptoms. Within this spectrum there is scope for increasingly empowering patients by involving them in decisions as they wish (Howie *et al.*, 1997). There is also scope for the preferred style of the patient and the clinician to match or clash. Depending on the nature of the decision and the preferences of the individuals concerned, it might be more or less easy and, indeed, comfortable to achieve agreement. However, outside the hospital setting, patients obviously control their medication use and have the final say, so it beholds clinicians to gain their support. The question is how and what to do if they can't.

A prescribing spectrum

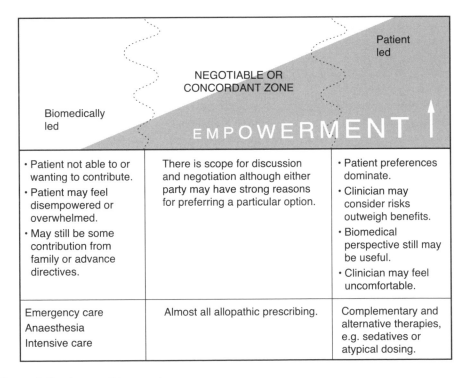

Figure 1.1 A prescribing spectrum.

Prescribing in a patient-centered way is therefore an approach designed to foster mutual understanding and collaboration. It does not imply that all patients should receive whatever they want. Clinicians have responsibilities to wider society as well as professional and institutional rules within which they must operate. How these factors can be managed when they conflict with patient-centered care is described in Chapter 7.

As most prescribing occurs in the primary healthcare setting, we make no apologies for the fact that much of our evidence and supporting case studies originates from family practice. To date this principally reflects interactions between doctors and patients, but nurses and pharmacists in both hospital and family practice are playing an increasing role in the prescribing process. Consequently, this book is aimed at all professionals involved in the process of helping patients to consider and use pharmaceutical products. We use the generic term 'clinician' throughout to include anyone playing this role in a pharmacy, family practice or hospital setting, and in Chapter 6 we discuss how different professionals can help patients to participate in the process even if they themselves do not prescribe.

The book is structured in two sections. The first section (Chapters 2, 3 and 4) considers what the literature tells us about medication use from the perspectives of the clinician, the patient and behavioral sciences, respectively. This more academic perspective is illustrated with numerous patients' stories and quotes, especially in Chapter 4, and is designed to provide the understanding required to interpret what patients are likely to say. The second section (Chapter 5 onwards) is a more practically orientated 'how to' guide, and for hasty clinicians who wish to skip the background material we would recommend Chapter 5 as the start of the more applied techniques for exploring individual patients' medication use and intervening in a patient-centered manner.

Chapter 2 commences by discussing the volume of medicines prescribed and some of the problems that appear to result from patients' responses, before exploring these issues from the medical perspective. We then move on to consider how medicines fit into patients' lives more broadly, how their views affect their decisions about medicines, and what this implies for the prescribing process. In Chapter 4, using research material from our own projects and from the available literature, we shall explore how various psychosocial models might help to explain medicine-taking behaviors and the implication of this for practice.

The second section of the book is aimed specifically at those with responsibility for prescribing. We present a potentially more manageable single model of the relevant factors developed through research based on both patients' experiences of receiving medicines and doctors' experiences of prescribing in a number of settings. By presenting patients' stories we hope to help clinicians to see how they can access patients' thinking about both illness and treatment. This is extended in Chapter 6 by considering how to develop more patient-centered approaches to the process of prescribing, under what we might term 'normal' conditions of clinical practice. It also considers how other professionals can assist or disrupt this process. Chapter 7 introduces techniques that have been devised from patient-centered principles to use when *non-compliance* is thought to be likely. Again, examples are given to illustrate the process. Chapter 8 presents some of the unresolved issues and highlights the difficult issues that can arise – for instance, when patient choice clashes with evidence-based approaches. The final chapter contains a synopsis of patient-centered prescribing, discusses some areas that merit further research and presents ideas about how you may seek to develop these skills if you wish to.

By the end of this book we hope that you, the reader, will have a good understanding of the current issues with regard to the prescribing process and medicine-taking behaviors. You should also be in a position to experiment with new approaches to prescribing medicines, based on a richer understanding of patients' thoughts, feelings and behaviors. You might do this in the hope of at least diffusing potentially difficult clinical relationships and sometimes significantly improving suboptimal patient care. And here, immediately, we strike upon one of the key issues for this whole concept. Is the goal always to improve what clinicians see as suboptimal care? Surely this is true when it accords with the patient's priorities, but what if it might not do so? Even assuming that we have overcome the difficulties of sharing information and can be confident that a decision is truly *informed*, when do a patient's values override clinical practice or protocols? Throughout this text, as we weave a course between patient autonomy and clinicians' responsibility, this line becomes as blurred as it is in practice. But, as authors, our stance is clear – it is the clinician's role to advise to the best of their abilities but not to dictate what patients should do unless they are explicitly invited to do so.

Definitions

The language surrounding medication use is often a sensitive matter, and it can obscure the issues if not handled consistently. It might therefore be helpful to clarify the way we have sought to address this problem and to indicate how we have chosen to use selected words. Although many readers will be very conscious of a preference for the term *adherence* over recent years, we have elected to use *compliance* throughout the text precisely because it highlights the paternalistic nature of the underlying assumptions that this concept reflects. This is not because we support the term, but rather because we want to highlight the incongruence of the concept unambiguously. Adhering to advice, even voluntarily, does not seem to be sufficiently distinct from complying with an instruction. Neither requires the patient to participate in or share the decisions that are made.

In order to provide a more considered approach, we clarify here how we are using these terms.

Compliance/adherence

This is the extent to which medication use follows the prescriber's instruction. This may be ideal, over or under that recommended, or vary in other ways such as timing, frequency of dosage or route of administration.

Compliant/adherent

This term describes a pattern of medication use that matches the prescriber's instruction. The extent to which use and instruction correspond may vary, but the acceptable level is determined by the clinician.

Concordance/patient-centered prescribing

Here there is agreement between the patient and the prescriber that a treatment is an effective way of achieving the patient's goals. It is characterized by an exchange of views designed to mutually inform each other, and a process of establishing a sufficiently shared decision. Agreement may be easy, may require negotiation or may possibly be agreement to differ, in which case the beliefs and wishes of the patient take priority. Discordance is not a judgemental term, as it does not favour either view. Hence non-concordance is a misnomer and is not in any way a synonym for *non-compliance*.

Discrepant medication use

This term is suggested to describe patterns of medication use that do not match those intended by the patient – for instance, due to low motivation or perhaps memory problems.

Medication use/actual use

This refers to the actual way in which a prescribed medicine is used, in terms of frequency, timing, route and dosage employed, irrespective of instructions or intentions.

Non-compliance/non-adherence

This occurs when any parameter of medication use varies from that advised or instructed. Research studies often use a cut-off value of 20% or more variance to define this (Morris and Schulz, 1992). This is independent of clinical outcome and may be categorized by the following:

- parameter – dose, frequency, timing, route
- extent – amount above or below recommended dose
- impact – dangerous vs. trivial
- intent – intentional vs. accidental
- disclosure – open vs. concealed.

Non-encashment

This occurs when a prescription is issued but not collected from a pharmacist. In such circumstances the medication cannot have been taken and may offer one way of estimating medication use.

Therapeutic coverage

This refers to the range of medication use which might be expected, from the pharmacokinetic viewpoint, to produce the desired effect with minimal risk (Meredith and Elliott, 1994).

Understanding the issues

Chapter 2

Taking medicines

David Snadden

Part 1: The burden of the problem

Introduction

In his letter to Jean Baptiste Le Roy in 1789, Benjamin Franklin said that 'In this world nothing can be said to be certain, except death and taxes.' It is worth pondering whether everyone will not, at some stage in their life, take some sort of medicine, be it a folk remedy or pharmaceutical product. Perhaps 'medicine taking' needs to be added to Franklin's statement to reflect an increasing reality of modern life.

But the process of providing medical care and its interaction with medication use is not straightforward, and has been a longstanding cause of friction, as illustrated by this extract from *The History and Statutes of the Royal Infirmary of Edinburgh* from 1778.

> Such patients are to be expelled from the infirmary: Who refuse the food, drink, medicines or operations prescribed or take any medicines, drink or food, not ordered by the physicians or surgeons.
>
> (Hugh Baron, 2004)

For those who doubt that the practice of medicine is changing, it might be useful to contrast this with the modern enthusiasm for encouraging patients not only to participate in healthcare decisions but also, on occasion, to insist upon their rights of autonomy. The balance of power has clearly shifted and continues to do so.

The size of the issue

The volume of prescribed medications consumed is huge. In Scotland in 1996–7, a total of 55 million items were prescribed for a population of just over 5 million, representing an average of 11 items per year per person at a cost of £492 million (Scottish Office, 1997). In 2002, expenditure on medicines ranged from 2.6% GDP (£437 per head) in the USA to 0.9% GDP (£116 per head) in Ireland (Association of the British Pharmaceutical Industry, 2005). Expenditure on medicines is increasing rapidly. In the USA it rose by 11% during 2003 to an estimated US$184 billion (Moynihan, 2004). Because clinicians believe in what they prescribe and want to achieve good results, and because society invests so much in medicines, there has been extensive research into the topic. For clinicians this has focussed on the application of evidence through a process of 'rational prescribing.' For patients it has tended to focus on the extent to which they have followed the prescribed regime – that is, the extent to which they have been *compliant*. Only recently has this begun to shift towards a more collaborative conceptualization which recognizes the need to balance clinicians' and patients' views more equally.

Clinicians' stories are laced with examples such as:

> Patient: *"I have just come in for my pills."*
> Doctor: *"From my computer here you don't seem to be getting through much of this ... I am a bit concerned ..."*
> Patient: *"Well actually, doctor, I find them a bit of a pest to take. They give me a bad tummy and I do 'forget' them sometimes."*

How should a patient-centered clinician respond?

Debugging 'compliance'

Traditional thinking tends to view medication use or misuse in terms of *compliance*. Compliance is usually defined in terms of whether an individual follows the prescriber's instructions. A common pragmatic definition of *non-compliance* is anyone taking more than 20% or less than 20% of the medicine as instructed (Morris and Schulz, 1992). Although dichotomous statements of *compliance/non-compliance* have to be based upon such crude classifications, this has many weaknesses and is unhelpful for many reasons. First, it generally takes no account of patterns and timing of consumption, let alone the way in which this accords with the pharmacokinetics of the preparation. More importantly, it takes no account of outcome. Even if it is assumed that favourable clinical outcomes correlate with high compliance, it cannot be assumed that this is the optimal outcome from the patient's perspective, as the above scenario implies. Of course clinicians are used to tailoring treatment according to side-effects, and this is seen as a legitimate patient contribution, but to what extent are the patient's views to be accepted?

Discussing how medicines are actually used is fascinating, as demonstrated by the following description by a doctor in her late forties, reporting her use of hormone replacement therapy (in 1990s):

> Well it is really odd, I can't stand the progesterone part as it makes me feel awful, I know I am meant to take it and I know it protects me from cancer and stuff like that, but I hate it so much I often don't bother and just take the oestrogen. After a few months I have great surges of guilt and either take the progesterone for too long, or even double it up for a while in the faint hope I can get the protective bit in as quick as possible. I know this is totally irrational, but that is what I do.

(All of the cases we cite come directly from our research work, but names and some details have been altered to protect anonymity without altering the substance of the meaning.)

Here we have a well-informed patient manipulating the way she uses her hormone replacement therapy to suit her symptoms and concerns best. Is this problematic *non-compliance* or is it patient-centered medication use? How should the prescriber respond?

The word 'compliance' is itself controversial. The *Oxford English Dictionary* defines *compliance* as 'obedience to a request or command.' Consequently it has long been criticized because of its authoritarian overtones and the implication that patients ought to do what a clinician tells them to do (Moore, 1988). As medicine is becoming less paternalistic, others prefer terms such as 'adherence' (Morris and Schulz, 1992). Although the definition of adherence is much the same ('follow in detail or give allegiance to'), it perhaps has less paternalistic overtones. However, both terms conceptually divorce medication use from the patient's experience, and professionals often appear to use compliance as a proxy for a successful outcome. So in this paradigm a successful clinician will manage to get patients to take the medicines they recommend in the way they advise in an effort to minimize symptoms or extend longevity as much as possible. The clinician is deemed to 'know best', and the patient's role is to apply their advice diligently.

However, there is a growing literature which suggests that patients do not share this view and that they place equal or greater value on personal and possibly competing goals (Morris and Schulz, 1993; Britten, 1994). They do not necessarily evaluate medicines primarily on the basis of their clinical effectiveness, but by how they affect their lives and fit in with their belief systems. Hence *non-compliance* may result from a patient's beliefs or goals for treatment differing from those of the clinician. Thus clinicians who try to deal with poor compliance using tactics like long dosing schedules, long-acting drugs, warning about risks or using memory aids may be missing the primary reason for drugs not being taken as directed. As patients are autonomous and as it is they who, at the end of the day, are being expected to swallow the pills, they will always have the final say. Consequently, as currently employed, both *compliance* and *adherence* are unhelpful terms which focus attention on the intermediate step of medication use rather than the patient's goals. However, lest this view be too heretical, we should acknowledge that modern pharmaceuticals are backed by considerable evidence that justifies clinicians bothering about how they are finally used. Rather, we are arguing that the patient's contribution to the prescribing process and consequent use of medicines has received too little attention and offers great potential to improve care.

At this point we should recognize that although compliance and adherence are not particularly helpful terms, we do need to be able to label and discuss different patterns of medication use. We have elected to use compliance to describe medication use that differs substantively (in a way likely to affect the clinical outcome) from that prescribed or directed by the prescriber, irrespective of the reason, which is often not known. This accords with the continuing common use of this phrase in medical practice. However, someone may rationally decide that they wish to take a medicine in a particular way, or indeed simply accept the prescriber's guidance but then fail to actually use the medicines as they intended for any of many reasons. We have termed this *discrepant* medication use. By definition this requires patients to have decided how to use the medicine and reflects what has also been described as 'unintentional' or 'accidental' *non-compliance*. We are seeking to separate the prescribing process and decision making from the process of consuming the medicine. So to explore things further, let us try to understand medication use in more detail. These terms will be *italicised* throughout the text to try to reinforce this distinction.

How researchers estimate whether people take drugs or not

One of the problems in monitoring medication use is that clinicians can rarely be sure whether patients take their drugs or not. There are basically three methods that have been used to try to measure this (Walker and Wright, 1985a,b; Pullar *et al.*, 1989):

1 self-reports using interviews or questionnaires
2 proxy markers such as pill counts and dispensing records
3 biochemical measurements.

Patient reports have proved least reliable and consistently indicate greater *compliance* when compared with any other method, although they can offer insights into patterns of use and patients' reasoning, and are convenient to use (Maenpaa *et al.*, 1987a,b; Tashkin *et al.*, 1991; Matsui *et al.*, 1994). Similarly, proxy markers such as prescription requests or dispensing also overestimate drug consumption, if to a lesser degree. Microchip devices have the potential to give information on the time when doses are taken or at least when bottles are opened, but are generally only available to researchers. However, crude proxy markers such as counting remaining pills or examining prescription records (to see how prescriptions issued or collected from pharmacies compare with treatment required) can be very useful in practice (Fletcher *et al.*, 1979; Rudd *et al.*, 1988). These proxy markers can give an accurate idea of drugs not taken, but cannot determine whether prescriptions collected or pills not in bottles were actually taken. Finally, there is a range of biochemical estimates available. These are probably the most accurate, but are rarely practical in the clinical situation due to individual variation in drug metabolism, the need for additional sampling and the expense involved. They rely on measurements of the drug or metabolite in blood or urine (Fletcher *et al.*, 1979; Maenpaa *et al.*, 1987a; Perel, 1988), the addition of tracer chemicals (Jay *et al.*, 1984; Roth *et al.*, 1996) or enzyme markers (Satterfield *et al.*, 1990). Interestingly, this research on *compliance* has focussed on establishing what medicines have been taken and when, not on how or why they were used, or on the patient's treatment goals. Perhaps as a result, some bizarre behavior has been reported and this has been used to suggest that patients often seek to mislead us about their medication use – for instance, concocting diary entries or wasting remaining doses from inhalers (fitted with electronic dose recording devices) (Tashkin *et al.*, 1991; Stone *et al.*, 2002). However, these behaviors may well be the result of the research process itself, which can create atypical responses, as participants may know that they are being studied and seek to appear compliant for that reason. Some researchers have managed to obtain highly accurate accounts that correlate well with biochemical markers, suggesting that much of this *compliance-focussed* research might not be relevant to a more collaborative clinical setting (Fletcher *et al.*, 1979; Satterfield *et al.*, 1990). This still leaves the following questions. To what extent are medicines used as the prescriber would wish? And does patients' use of medicines matter in terms of clinical outcomes?

What proportion of medication is taken?

There is a vast literature describing the extent to which patients are consistently found not to take their medicines as directed. This universal phenomenon appears to affect all conditions and populations (Walker and Wright, 1985a,b). Probably the largest review of this topic concluded that only around half of all medicines are taken appropriately (Haynes *et al.*, 1996). Of course this is highly dependent upon the way the term 'appropriate' is defined, which varies between studies. A more recent review analysed studies published between 1996 and 2002 and concluded that there is overwhelming evidence that *non-compliance* continues to be a universal problem in all 14 disease groups which they reported separately (Carter *et al.*, 2003). It is a particular problem with preventive treatments, but also applies in life-threatening conditions such as cancer therapies and transplant recipients, as well as in symptomatic conditions such as depression and arthritis.

Compliance in different conditions

Table 2.1 Compliance in different conditions

Condition	Range of mean compliance reported (%)	Number of studies
Diabetes	57	1
Epilepsy	65–86	3
Leprosy	24–85	7
Oral contraceptives	45–62	2
Peptic ulcer disease	47–54	3
Psychiatric problems	38–86	5
Tuberculosis	43–93	3

Source: Walker and Wright (1985b).

Although the nature of the individual or the condition appears to have relatively little impact on the likelihood of medicines being used effectively, the need for convenient dosing has been consistently reported.

Compliance rate by dosage schedule

Table 2.2 Compliance rate by dosage schedule

Dosage Schedule	Compliance	
	Range (%)	Mean ± SEM (%)
Once daily	42–93	73 ± 6
Twice daily	50–94	70 ± 5
Three times daily	18–89	52 ± 7
Four times daily	11–66	42 ± 5

Source: Greenburg (1984).
SEM, standard error of mean.

Does taking medicine improve health outcomes?

In general the effect of a drug is assessed by its impact on mortality, morbidity, relevant clinical markers and measures such as admission rates (Sclar and Pharm, 1991;

Chewning and Sleath, 1996; McGrae *et al.*, 1997). Not surprisingly, there is good evidence gathered over many years that taking medicines in the doses recommended does improve health outcomes. For example, taking anti-tuberculosis drugs properly does reduce positive TB cultures (Fox, 1983a,b), taking drugs that lower blood pressure actually produces better blood pressure control (Logan *et al.*, 1979; McKenney *et al.*, 1992), and blood pressure readings have also been shown to correlate with number of pills swallowed (Meyer *et al.*, 1985). Similar findings have been described in diabetes, where non-compliant young adults had worse control and were admitted to hospital more frequently (Morris *et al.*, 1997), with aspirin use following femoro-popliteal bypass surgery (Franks *et al.*, 1992), and in primary prevention of myocardial infarction (Glynn *et al.*, 1994). So the evidence suggests that medicines really do improve clinical outcomes when used appropriately.

However, there is very little in the literature that evaluates medication use in relation to patient satisfaction, preferences, quality-of-life markers and even more patient-centered outcomes such as a patient-generated index (Ruta *et al.*, 1994). Clearly patients do not take medicines in the way that clinicians wish, but to some extent this could be because they prioritize different outcomes and operate according to different beliefs. Perhaps they do not want to take the medicines as prescribed, rather than being unable to. This is not a new problem, and one study in the early 1970s found that around 75% of patients consumed 80% of the drugs prescribed, but that this consumption rate fell to 64% when they had any doubts about the treatment – for instance, if they did not think it was necessary, if the dose was too high or the treatment too long, or if no improvement occurred (Dunnel and Cartwright, 1972).

So it is clear that there is a real missed opportunity, because many potent pharmaceutical products are not being used in a way that is likely to maximize the benefits which they were designed to provide. However, the medical focus of researchers appears not to have been balanced well by work exploring patients' views and values. Others have drawn similar conclusions. For instance, one large and well-designed study examined outcomes over 4 years in 2,125 patients with high blood pressure, diabetes, recent myocardial infarction or heart failure. The investigators summarized their findings as follows: *"We cannot conclude that assisting patients with these conditions to adhere to their physician's recommendations will necessarily lead to better health over time"* (Hays *et al.*, 1994). Haynes and colleagues, who are leading authors on this topic, also conclude in their systematic review that there is little irrefutable evidence to support any intervention, that potentially large benefits are being missed, and that innovative, fundamental and applied research is still required (Haynes *et al.*, 1996). Alarmingly, this conclusion is no advance upon the thorough review and recommendations of Meichenbaum and Turk published in 1987, so there appears to be an impasse. Clinicians do not know how to get patients to take their treatments as directed, and although doing so would improve clinical outcomes, we cannot be confident that other problems of equal importance to patients would not be created.

Perhaps we should be thinking more broadly and not considering medication use as a rational, cognitive process primarily amenable to logical argument or persuasion. If so, we might assume that patients would comply with drug treatment for serious conditions, as in many ways their lives depend on it. Even here the available evidence suggests that there is more to medicine taking than meets the professional eye or assumption. A third of children in remission from leukaemia fail to take sufficient treatment, and even post transplant surgery *non-compliance* is common (3–50% of cases) and associated with rejection (Lilleyman and Lennard, 1996; Laederach-Hofmann and Bunzel, 2000). At the very least, clinicians might want to take account of the reservations that patients commonly express about taking medicines. Many feel ambivalent about using pharmaceutical products and have reservations about medicines in general, as well as concerns and ideas about their own treatments (Horne and Weinman, 1999; Townsend *et al.*, 2003).

Case example: Jane

Jane is an asthmatic woman who is continually attempting to reduce the amount of inhaled steroid she consumes, despite the fact that she knows this medication improves her condition. She believes in 'fighting' her condition, and managing with minimal treatment is part of this. For her, more treatment implies greater illness, not better care.

> Jane: "It's just the way I've been brought up by my dad, like I said, it's just always fight it. He's never … it's just his attitude you never give in to anything, if you can help take as little as you can if you can get away with it."
> Interviewer: "So would … would taking it, you know, regularly twice a day, would that be giving in?"
> Jane: "Well, yeah, in his eyes yeah."
> Interviewer: "What about your eyes?"
> Jane: "If I'm bad, no. Well, in the summer when I'm feeling OK I say what's the point, 'cause I feel fine. It's hard to explain. If you're feeling good you don't need to depend on them. I think it's just having to depend on something all your life day in day out."
> Interviewer: "You've mentioned this word lots of times but this is you isn't it, this is part of your character, this 'fight' against your asthma?"
> Jane: "Oh always. It's just the way my dad's brought me up 'cause he lost his brother through asthma, he had a bad heart attack through asthma so since then he's always told everybody to fight it. … So I think it gives you more of a chance if you're willing to fight what you've got."

Patients' use of drugs has also been looked at as a factor precipitating hospital admission, with one study suggesting that 5.5% of all hospital admissions in the USA were primarily attributed to *non-compliance* (Sullivan *et al.*, 1990). However, this study omitted to estimate drug reactions if *compliance* increased, which have been estimated as causing up to 17% of all admissions for the elderly (Sclar and Pharm, 1991). So perhaps health professionals have been slow to acknowledge the drawbacks of *compliance* in terms of costs as well as benefits. If we add this finding to some strong but puzzling evidence from well-designed trials that substantial benefits are gained through complying with placebo treatments (even in terms of *hard* effects such as reduced mortality following myocardial infarction) (Coronary Drug Project Research Group, 1980; Horwitz and Horwitz, 1993; Glynn *et al.*, 1994), we might be left wondering whether the status quo is not about 'as good as it gets.'

This is probably a slightly heretical statement, as the balance of evidence suggests that taking medicines does improve health outcomes, even if some of this benefit is a placebo effect and there are drawbacks such as side-effects and some ambivalence for many patients to overcome. Perhaps the main conclusion to be drawn from this conflicting evidence is that medicine taking is an area fraught with problems, that it is difficult to research, and that the clinician and patient often appear to have different agendas. These agendas have not, at least in terms of the body of research evidence, been explored in a way that allows us to suggest how clinicians and patients can work together to define and search for optimal outcomes.

Societal changes from paternalistic to participative medicine

The role of medicine and medication needs to be set in a wider societal context. Certainly in western medicine doctors have until recently been seen to be paternalistic, often handing down treatments and remedies to patients with little explanation or perceived need for understanding on the patient's part. Perhaps this is not surprising, as only recently has medicine had really effective (and justifiable) medicines and technical interventions at its disposal. For example, the widespread availability of antibiotics has only come about in the last 50 years or so, yet now this is taken for granted to the point where antibiotics are abused and antibiotic resistance is a growing problem. As society becomes more open, as information becomes more readily available to all and as various laws make information a right for individuals, we are gradually moving towards a situation where more open contracts need to be established between clinicians and patients. It is likely that such openness can only be founded on trust and open information sharing on both sides. This gradual shift has led to the development of various consulting models that attempt to put the patient at the heart of the consultation. These models encourage the clinician to understand not only the disease, but also how it affects the patient and how the patient's life, family, work and health beliefs affect the progress of their illness and their view of the treatment options (Pendleton *et al.*, 1984; Stewart *et al.*, 1995). This may be seen as a maturing of the clinical relationship, with patients no longer being treated in a childlike fashion and being told what to do by paternalistic professionals, but having the option of participating in decisions on a more equal basis. This increased freedom comes with additional responsibility, of course, and this is a theme that we shall revisit later.

So we know that pharmaceuticals play a crucial role in modern care, but that medicine-taking behaviors are complex and not yet comprehensively understood. There appears to be considerable lost opportunity because of suboptimal treatment use, but it is not clear how this can be effectively remedied or, indeed, if the anticipated benefits would really result if this could be done. The existing research has failed to resolve this issue satisfactorily, and meanwhile society is changing in a way that requires a change in the traditional relationships between patients and their healthcare professionals. This suggests that we need to work on how we talk to people, how we understand them, and how we establish new ways of talking about medicines and promote more open consultations. These ideas are discussed in greater depth in Chapters 6 and 7.

Understanding complex social phenomena

From a philosophical perspective, modern medicine is founded on and remains largely driven by reductionist science. Medicine's huge advances are considered to be based predominantly on measurement and experimentation. This philosophy suggests that by deconstructing complex systems and experimenting with the components, we should be able to understand the whole. For example, drugs that lower blood pressure have been developed from an experimental understanding of physiology, biochemistry and pathology. This approach allows us to understand cause and effect and to predict the impact of treatments on an individual.

Despite the enormous strengths of the experimental approach, it has some weaknesses. One problem is that experimental science is based on the concept of universal truth. What is seen to be true in one experimental situation is also believed to be true in other similar settings. In other words, the finding can be generalized to relevant populations. However, this assumption may be less reliable when considering human behaviors, especially the behaviors of individuals which may be influenced by social factors that cannot be controlled for or perhaps even measured – for instance, having a fear of treatment. Behaviors are more difficult to study using experimental methods than are body systems.

In pharmacokinetic experiments, confounding variables may be tightly controlled. To achieve this, a medication for high blood pressure might not be tested for its effect on people with multiple problems, as this might confuse interpretation of the results and complicate the study. Indeed many major trials have been conducted using solely male participants, or those under 75 years of age. Although this makes for cleaner experiments, it causes problems in the messy world of clinical practice as our patients frequently have multiple problems, or are from groups that were excluded from trials. Hence we should be cautious when generalising findings. Evidence from trials may be very difficult to apply to individuals. For instance, side-effects, the likelihood of which may be assessed as rare according to the percentage of people affected in large trials, suddenly become crucial when dealing with a unique individual who experiences or believes him- or herself to be at risk of suffering a particular effect.

Experimental science also cannot explain phenomena like the placebo effect, mentioned above, or the effect of personal and social beliefs on illness and outcomes. For instance, diabetic control in adolescent populations in two European cities (one in Italy and the other in Scotland) was found to be quite different despite similar healthcare structures and guidelines governing recommended care. No quantified data could explain this. However, a qualitative study of the process of care in the two settings revealed that increased family involvement and social support structures in the Italian culture appear to promote better healthcare outcomes in this age group (Greene, 2001). These limitations of the experimental method may also explain our limited understanding about how and why people take medicines as they do. While we have concentrated on the causes of disease and the effect of medicines, the human factor has been relatively ignored. In other words, we have not researched the phenomenon of medicine taking at all broadly and, in particular, we have researched the patients' perspective very little.

The researching of processes, beliefs and related phenomena needs a different approach, and the social sciences can help us to understand these more human factors. It is therefore no accident that much of the research presented later in this book is based on interpretive studies using qualitative methods. These seek to understand the complex beliefs and behaviors that people demonstrate with regard to their medicines and during related consultations. Only by understanding these can we help to translate the huge strides that medicine has made for the optimal benefit of patients. Those who prescribe drugs therefore need to know as much about how an individual patient views and intends to use a drug as they do about the pathological and pharmacological processes involved. Blending these components is the real 'art' of medicine. If they are to produce good art, this book will argue, practitioners need some new tools to help to disentangle the complexities which we have outlined above. These tools are largely encompassed within the framework of the patient-centered clinical method, although we suggest a number of ways in which their use may be refined in the context of problematic medication use.

Dispensing with the 'problem' of compliance

Part of the difficulty with the concept of *compliance* is that this pejorative idea hinders our understanding. The term now has enormously negative overtones and, in the era of patient participation, a touch of autocracy. If we wish to argue for finding new ways for clinicians and patients to understand each other – and we do – then we have to dispense with such overtones. We need to recognize that patients are no longer (on the whole) passive, and that consultations are increasingly becoming more of a 'meeting between experts' (Tuckett *et al.*, 1985). We also need to think in terms of what we mean by successful therapy. We need to consider what a good outcome for a patient is. Often the clinical outcome will be the main priority for the patient, but there may be much more to it than that. We need to learn to negotiate in order to find the most acceptable ways of helping patients to achieve their health goals, and we need to understand how medicines might be used as a result. A number of alternatives to the notion of *compliance* have been suggested, and the one that is gaining most favour at the moment is the term *concordance* (Blenkinsopp *et al.*, 1997). Concordance represents an agreement between prescriber and patient that a treatment is the most likely way of achieving their shared goals. In other words, it implies an interaction that respects the beliefs and wishes of the patient. This is about achieving a meeting of minds in an adult-style relationship, which means that the conclusion may not match the recommended guidelines on prescribing practice. And, of course, it remains inevitable that actual medication use will still vary somewhat from the agreed use.

This notion may be scary for clinicians, for as patients get to have a greater say about their medicines, we might have to understand why they don't want to take them and we might have to agree to pharmacologically suboptimal use that contravenes current clinical guidelines. It might also mean giving a patient permission to use drugs in a way that we might not feel too comfortable about, with all the associated legal and ethical difficulties that this might bring. It really means a whole new way of thinking about and talking to patients about how they use their medicines – this is the ultimate conclusion of patient-centered care. Many clinicians already involve patients in decisions about treatment, and many patients already insist on influencing decisions even when this option is not offered. The difference here is that the balance of power is being explicitly offered to patients, even in situations when harm may result. Indeed it is argued that doing this can be instrumental in resolving tense or even acrimonious relationships, and can produce improvements even in the face of apparently intransigent views.

Part 2: The medical perspective

In the second half of this chapter we shall consider some of the issues presented by the prescribing process from a clinician's point of view. We shall examine aspects of medicine-taking behaviors and how doctors have tried to improve them. We shall also touch upon some of the ethical dilemmas that are presented by developments such as clinical standards, guidelines and algorithms.

Case example

Let's start with a doctor/patient dialogue. Susan Green is a woman in her late forties who has suffered from asthma for years. This visit follows a recent hospital admission that included a respiratory arrest in an ambulance. Here we present the doctor and patient with two voices – the spoken and the hidden.

> Dr Rogers: "I thought I ought to drop by about your asthma as it seems you had a difficult time in hospital." ["The hospital told me you nearly died and I am jolly glad you got there on time."]
> Susan: "Yes, I felt pretty grim, but I am OK now." ["Oh no, here we go again – another lecture on my drugs coming up."]
> Dr Rogers: "Tell me what drugs you are taking now." ["I know her compliance is a problem. The computer shows she cannot be using enough steroids, but perhaps this has been sorted whilst she was in hospital."]
> Susan: "Well, pretty much the same as before, you know the blue one and the brown one, both inhalers." ["I still really don't know what these do, but everyone presumes I do, and I feel stupid asking after all this time. I don't think the brown one makes the slightest difference."]
> Dr Rogers: "Well, are you taking them OK?" ["I've told her so many times what they are for and when to take them it seems pointless going over this again, but I don't want to have another experience like this one."]
> Susan: "Well, yes, just the way I have always done." ["I am really scared I am going to die next time."]
> Dr Rogers: "Look, you were so sick this time I cannot emphasize enough that you really must take these as you've been told to." ["I wonder if she really does take them."]
> Susan: "Well, I do." ["I'm confused. They keep telling me to take drugs that make no difference, and I can't really discuss it because I keep saying I do take them. I'll look silly."]
> Dr Rogers: "Well, that's OK then." [I'll just have to give a prescription now and see what happens."]

This patient has suffered several life-threatening asthmatic episodes. She attends asthma clinics and is prescribed large doses of preventive (steroid) and relieving drugs which her doctors are convinced she does not take properly. As her asthma attacks have been severe and fast to develop, they dread her calls, which have previously meant managing an alarmingly sick patient and providing emergency treatment before transfer to hospital, where she has required mechanical ventilation. Let us examine the above dialogue to see what is going on.

Both doctor and patient appear to be scared of the same thing – the patient dying. Neither voices this at the time, but both make assumptions. The patient assumes that the doctor will be upset that she still doesn't understand or use her medicines well, and the doctor assumes that he doesn't need to tell her again as she has been told so often. There is a feeling that both are sitting on a powder keg and neither knows how to deal with it. The situation is emotionally charged for both parties. We shall return to this patient's story later in the book, as the outcome is fascinating, but for now let us explore the traditional medical perspective on this type of problem.

The treatment of asthma is laid down quite clearly in various guidelines on the treatment and prevention of asthma in the UK, Canada, the USA, Australia and elsewhere. These state how incremental steps should be followed if the condition is not controlled. They also advocate that patients are monitored regularly, including how and when they use their medication. In addition, the guidelines emphasize the importance of patient education to ensure that they know what the medicines are for, how the medicines should be used, and what to do if their condition deteriorates.

There is no doubt that applying evidence-based medicine through the application of clinical guidelines can improve patient care, but implementing guidelines in practice appears to be very difficult. Most attempts have met with very limited success (Grimshaw and Russell, 1993; Grilli and Lomas, 1994). Perhaps the above dialogue helps to illustrate why this might be and also indicates a way forward. Guidelines are refined clinical algorithms, and are therefore focussed on clinical measures and endpoints. They leave no space for the 'hidden voices' which, perhaps partly as a result of this, are rarely heard. This approach to patient care – which privileges medical knowledge above the patient's perspective – fails to acknowledge the crucial role that the patient's views and beliefs can have. This book series, and indeed the whole shift towards a more 'patient-centered' approach to medical care, seeks to redress this balance. Not only does the patient's voice need to be heard in terms of their ideas, concerns and expectations about the diagnosis, but it also needs to be used to help to formulate a treatment plan that the patient feels they own and want to implement. This is not reflected in the bulk of the research into medication use in the medical literature.

Clinicians' perceptions of why patients take medicines in the way they do

Looking at the medical literature on medication use, there are a number of themes that have been explored to explain why patients may not take medicines in the way that they are advised. These fall into four general categories, namely patient factors, professional characteristics, medicine effects, and the nature of the condition.

Patient factors

Many studies have sought demographic variables associated with *non-compliance* such as age, gender, level of education, etc., in order to determine which individuals are likely to be *non-compliant*, but this has not proved helpful. One review of over 100 articles concluded:

> Inconsistent findings, which do not transfer between different disease conditions, have made it impossible to develop a prototype of a non-compliant individual. More than 20 years of research has produced very little consistent information on the factors which can be correlated with non-compliant behaviour.
>
> (Morris and Schulz, 1992)

Another review concludes:

> Every patient is a potential defaulter. In short, non-adherence can be a problem for any population.
>
> (Meichenbaum and Turk, 1987)

It might also be helpful to consider whether patients might intentionally not take medicines or accidentally omit them. Two studies (Begg, 1984; Beardon *et al.*, 1993) have shown that around 6% of prescriptions issued in the UK are not even collected from the pharmacy. This suggests a fundamental lack of agreement between clinician and patient about the conclusion of the consultation. A qualitative study that interviewed such patients reported four main reasons for not collecting their prescriptions (Jones and Britten, 1998):

1 the medicine was cheaper to buy over the counter
2 the clinician had given the patient *permission* not to take it
3 the patient had an unhelpful understanding of their illness
4 some were seeking to maintain control over their care.

Other patients interviewed in an earlier study by Fletcher and colleagues gave more conventional explanations for not taking digoxin. These included forgetfulness, inconvenience, perceived side-effects and a feeling that the drug was no longer needed (Fletcher *et al.*, 1979). In one more recent study of elderly patients commencing a new medication, one third of the participants admitted to being *non-compliant*, and in half of these cases this was intentional (Barber *et al.*, 2004).

However, patients might also not take their medicine unintentionally. This could be because they misunderstand how they are meant to take the medicine, it may be because the therapeutic regime is too difficult to implement (Greenberg, 1984), the patient may have memory problems or, with a busy life, they may simply forget. This is not surprising when you consider that only about half of medical instructions regarding treatment can be recalled by patients on leaving their consultation (Ley, 1988). So there is a wide range of reasons why patients may not follow prescribed instructions. Some appear quite logical, others are amenable to further information and some, such as a need for control, are perhaps more complex.

To illustrate this, let us go back to Susan, the asthmatic whose case study was presented at the beginning of this section. The data here come from interviews with the patient, and from her medical records and discussions with her doctors. Following an extended research interview it transpired that Susan was not taking her medicines as directed, just as her doctors suspected. She was using her relieving medicines regularly and her preventive medicines when she felt bad. This was a puzzle, as for more than 10 years her records included numerous reports that she had been 'given' education and advice on how to use her medications. The key appears to be in the use of words like 'given.' The message might have been sent but it certainly hadn't been received, and this had not been recognized or addressed. This discovery suggests that an alternative and careful attempt to provide a more helpful understanding about the patient's condition might be a worthwhile investment.

Even when there are simple problems such as poor understanding, it will help if the professional can try to think him- or herself into the patient's position and see what the problem really feels like to them. While it is tempting to blame patients for defaulting, we need to understand their perspective before leaping to our own conclusions.

Professional characteristics

The evidence is mixed concerning the impact that practitioners have on how patients use their medicines. For example, in primary care in the UK it has been found that prescriptions are less likely to be collected from the pharmacy if they were issued by a doctor in training (Beardon *et al.*, 1993). However, two other studies suggested that there was little association between a variety of doctor characteristics and the outcome of illnesses or the taking of medicines (DiMatteo *et al.*, 1993; Winefield *et al.*, 1995). Specifically, they reported that practitioner characteristics such as age, gender and experience were not related to medicine taking.

However, there are a number of studies which demonstrate that communication (providing information, expressing affect and using a patient-centered style) can influence not only patient satisfaction but also both medication use and illness outcomes (Stewart, 1995; Williams *et al.*, 1998). For instance, Lassen found that six components of the consultation were associated with an intention to comply (Lassen, 1991):

1 expectations of the consultation
2 ideas about the health problem
3 contents of advice
4 explanation of the advice
5 patient's perception of quality of advice
6 perceived barriers to *compliance*.

However, the benefits of such patient-centered approaches do not seem to hold true all the time, with some patients appearing to prefer a directive style and other reviews concluding that the link between clinicians' style and outcomes is tenuous (Mead and Bower, 2002). One fascinating study compared the effect of giving placebo versus no medication along with a positive versus uncertain consultation style for minor illness. The style of consultation had a considerable effect, favouring a confident or more directive approach, more so than the use of a placebo (Thomas, 1987). Thus there is apparently contradictory evidence that both patient-centered and directive consultation styles can have benefits. If the style of the clinician is so important, how do we assess whether a medicine is working? Alternatively, being patient-centered may require the clinician to be directive, depending on the circumstances (Gore and Ogden, 1998).

Perhaps this confusion is not surprising. If you reflect on your own or your family's healthcare experiences, there will probably have been times when you wanted to think things through and discuss the options when there was a difficult decision to make, perhaps about a long-term medicine or the benefits of surgery. However, there may also have been times when the situation was overwhelming or the right treatment seemed so obvious that you simply wanted things to be sorted out with minimal discussion. Few if any of the studies included in the reviews cited above distinguished participants on this type of basis (their preference for a particular role on the occasion in question), so the heterogeneous mix of the study populations might be expected to complicate the findings, and runs the risk of failing to detect a clinically important effect.

So it would appear that clinician characteristics don't play much of a part in determining whether patients take their medicines or not, but how the clinician behaves during the consultation might do so. To obtain the best results you may have to be able to adapt your style to suit the individual and the circumstances. As if the practice of medicine isn't hard enough already, this makes the task of the clinician seem yet more daunting.

However, there may be hope in the form of 'shared decision making', to which we shall return later.

Before we leave the impact of professionals on medicine taking we should reiterate that it is not just doctors who are involved, and that the processes of healthcare can contribute to how medicines are taken. For example, pharmacists are well placed to support medicines being taken effectively, although the evidence gathered from specific research interventions with pharmacists suggests that their impact is also patchy (Hawe and Higgins, 1990; Sclar *et al.*, 1991). Nurses managing blood pressure in the workplace have been found to reach target levels of blood pressure better than doctors and to have more patients who are taking their medicines (Logan *et al.*, 1979). In conditions such as asthma and diabetes there has been a shift towards guided self-management, which includes educating patients better and giving them more control over their treatment. This has been shown to reduce asthma symptoms, emergency medical care and costs (Hoskins *et al.*, 1999; Lahdensuo, 1999). So not only should doctors and other healthcare professionals consider how they behave, but paying attention to the details of the care process might also pay dividends in terms of how people take medicines.

Medicine effects

Healthcare professionals have considered in great detail how medicines themselves affect drug use. A range of factors appear to be relevant, including the regime and the perceived benefits and drawbacks in terms of side-effects, costs, etc.

The frequency of dosage regimes appears to be consistently important. Most of these studies have used event-monitoring devices to estimate consumption, and it appears that there is little difference when once or twice daily dosing is used, but that consumption falls off with more frequent doses (Greenberg, 1984; Peterson *et al.*, 1984; Cramer, 1989). There is a further problem in that patients who take many medicines are also less likely to take them as prescribed (Haynes *et al.*, 1977). This would seem logical in that frequent dosage regimes and complicated ones are more difficult to take as instructed.

It would also seem logical that medication use would be influenced by the result of treatment. So we would expect that medicines are more likely to be used when the patient feels a therapeutic benefit, while those who perceive side-effects may take less medicine. This is borne out by research which indicates that symptom reduction enhances medication use (Meyer *et al.*, 1985), while people are more likely to stop taking medicines if they experience side-effects (Anastasio *et al.*, 1994; SIA Ltd, 1995). Costs are another factor, with prescriptions being less likely to be collected if patients have to pay for the medicine (Beardon *et al.*, 1993; Lundberg *et al.*, 1998).

In most situations the ideal drug would be 100% effective, with no side-effects, free and delivered in a single dose. Effective therapy would surely be easier if this was available, but whilst the pharmaceutical industry continues to develop ever cleaner products, clinicians and patients are left balancing their options. They must decide whether the benefits outweigh the drawbacks, although this is surely a very subjective matter that will depend on both the way in which symptoms are perceived and the values that are ascribed to them. A degree of gastrointestinal upset may be tolerable for some patients but not for others, yet it may prompt a clinician to change treatment if it is thought to herald a bleeding ulcer. Again, however, it is the patient's perception and values that should determine the outcome.

Nature of the condition

Finally, and perhaps surprisingly, the patient's condition seems to have no bearing on whether medicines are taken or not. It might be expected that medicines would be used more consistently in life-threatening or serious conditions, but research continually refutes this. From the contraceptive pill to TB, diabetes or post transplant surgery, it remains a common concern (Walker and Wright, 1985a,b; Morris *et al.*, 1997; Talbot *et al.*, 1998; Laederach-Hofmann and Bunzel, 2000; Maher *et al.*, 2003).

This evidence merely highlights earlier statements in this chapter that medicine taking is a very complex issue. Although paying attention to dosage regimes, careful explanation and patient education may have an impact, it would seem that healthcare workers need to look much more broadly at the relationship between patients and their medicines in order to understand how to support them more effectively. This might be more about understanding them as people in terms of their aspirations, beliefs and feelings as much as anything. To obtain a glimpse of the potential value of doing so, let us return to Susan Green's story.

Case example: Susan (continued)

In the last part of Susan's story it was implied that she managed her condition better once she and her doctor had reached an understanding of how the drugs worked. But there was a little more to it than this.

Susan lived in a fairly dusty rural cottage and had several horses which she enjoyed exercising until she became too wheezy to risk this activity. She very much wanted to be able to exercise them again.

Her doctors became increasingly frustrated with her as they thought that her horses, the other pets and considerable dust in her house were affecting her health. They reacted by becoming more directive with regard to what she must do and what medication she must take, and more threatening about the consequences of not doing so – potential death.

Both parties were scared of the same thing, but were not reacting to it in a trusting or collaborative way. In fact trust had fallen to such a low level that Susan asked for the tape to be turned off while she discussed her experiences (hence we cannot give a quote). Only once her previously unspoken fear had been discussed could some education about asthma occur and a joint course of action be agreed. This was the key that unlocked the conversation about medication use and produced a subsequent significant improvement in her condition. Not only did her breathing improve, with a reduction in acute attacks, but also her condition improved sufficiently for her to be able to resume contact with her horses.

This illustrates the value of sharing and understanding a patient's perspective at a deeper level, which will be one of the main focuses of later chapters. How and when might clinicians begin to approach consultations like this? Before we conclude this chapter we need to highlight some of the constraints, particularly ethical ones, that clinicians are faced with.

Conflict between patient-centered prescribing and clinical responsibility

So far this chapter has presented a rosy picture of predictable success and minimal difficulty in expanding the patient-centered ethos into even the most testing circumstances. Clearly this is not the reality that most clinicians face daily, and it is important to consider the problems it can present as well as those it can solve. The sceptical reader may wish to turn straight to Chapter 8 where these are discussed in more detail, before deciding whether the techniques described are ones they would wish to employ. Here we shall just highlight the potential difficulties so that the reader is aware of them from the outset and knows they will be discussed later along with suggested solutions.

First, *it takes two to tango*. To develop a successful collaborative therapeutic relationship requires input from both parties. This can be especially difficult if there are entrenched behaviors such as a deferent patient or concealed *non-compliance*. Although patients should be able to play a passive role and let their clinician advise them if they wish, more commonly this appears to occur by default rather than after careful consideration. Changing this can be difficult for both parties.

Secondly, the balance between patient-centered and evidence-based care may be difficult to strike and may make clinicians feel very vulnerable (Stewart *et al.*, 2003). Modern medicine has come to be dominated by the evidence-based practice movement (see www.ceppc.org/guidelines among many others). In many ways this has been a necessary attempt to ensure that clinical decisions are based on the best research evidence available so that patients receive the best treatment for their condition. However, guidelines can be difficult to fit to an individual patient. It is impossible to predict who will respond in an average or extreme manner to a therapy, and matching values and preferences to the evidence is a complex task.

Thirdly, there is a range of potential ethical and legal dilemmas that may arise. Patient autonomy is usually a simple matter, but not if the patient's competence is questionable. Some patients make requests for treatment that might be seen as unreasonable – either on grounds of cost or because it may be considered poor care. How can clinicians defend themselves from accusations of providing poor care when they are seeking to blend their view of best care with that of the patient? For clinicians, in a litigation-conscious age, this is potentially a very uncomfortable position in which to be.

Fourthly, there are a number of pragmatic issues that need to be considered. When is it appropriate to invest extra time to achieve a more patient-centered, collaborative decision? And how can decisions that deviate from standard practice be defended (both legally if necessary and, more commonly, from colleagues attempting to get them back to a more conventional approach)? What level of understanding is required before a clinician can justifiably claim that the patient made an informed choice and how might this be recorded?

Finally, it must be questioned to what extent society wants to invest in providing a patient-centered care process, of which prescribing is just one component. How far should individual freedom to request or even demand care that an individual perceives to be the best for them be allowed? What financial costs, healthcare workers' time and risks are acceptable? For instance, what risks to others are acceptable because an individual with an infectious disease declines treatment? Or is patient-centered prescribing only to be seen as another tool for attempting to 'get people to take their drugs', simply a subtle form of paternalistic manipulation?

We hope we have indicated here that medicine needs to learn to more consciously tread a delicate path between the rationalists who develop guidelines and measure health gain using only 'hard outcomes', and the artists who work in the incompletely understood and complex world of human behavior, beliefs and aspirations. This sentiment is summed up neatly in Mencken's Metalaw:

> For every human problem, there is a neat, simple solution; and it is always wrong.
>
> (Mencken, 1880–1956)

So is individualized patient care any better?

Now that we have highlighted the problems, let us also look at the potential of adapting the prescribing process to each individual. Is there evidence that this can improve care or even health outcomes?

Case example: Susan (continued)

Let us return to Susan again and consider what made the difference to her health. She had been given appropriate medicines, and had previously been supplied with lots of information, leaflets and advice by many people in a range of settings. Yet she didn't take her medicines as advised, and almost certainly as a result of this her life was threatened on a number of occasions. What appeared to improve this alarming situation was not more information but a doctor understanding her aspirations, expectations and fears, and acknowledging the relevance of these for her asthma management. Taking her views, beliefs and emotional responses into account had a dramatic effect despite the fact that there was no substantive change in the treatment that was 'prescribed.'

Now is this single narrative a hint that there are different ways to approach medicine-taking problems? There has already been much research that has tested ways of improving patient *compliance*, so why should this be different? One reason is that these studies have tended to use *compliance* as a goal – rather than outcomes related to health gain. Why should patients 'comply'? However, there is also considerable research that has used clinical endpoints, and we shall concentrate on that work here, although even this has focussed primarily on clinical outcomes, and patient preferences have rarely been assessed. This is a problem because the 'clinical goal' has been assumed to reflect success, which might not reflect patients' values. Therefore when interpreting this evidence we have to acknowledge that, just like guidelines, it assumes that all patients seek the normal or representative outcome and that the outcome which clinicians deem ideal is of principal importance to patients. Despite this, it is still helpful to see whether interventions that seek to alter how medicines are taken are effective, to assess which offer most potential. These studies fall into five areas:

- patient education
- treatment prompts
- convenience aids
- incentives
- counselling and enhanced communication interventions.

There is little convincing evidence from a number of studies on patient education (Colcher and Bass, 1972; Sackett *et al.*, 1975; Morisky *et al.*, 1983) that simple education or provision of information makes much difference to treatment use.

Treatment prompts such as bottles that flash or bleep when a pill is due to be taken (McKenney *et al.*, 1992), monthly reminders to attend a pharmacy for a medicine review (Sclar and Skaer, 1991), and blood pressure monitoring by self-recording or nurse visits have all been shown to improve health outcomes. This suggests that treatment prompts do improve medication use, although they are complex to set up and manage consistently. Similarly, convenience aids seem to be helpful for those patients who have difficulty organising their treatments, primarily the elderly, as suggested by a study on the use of blister packs (Wong and Norman, 1987). For more able patients, neither 28-day pill reminder packs nor combination asthma inhalers made a difference to health outcomes (Becker *et al.*, 1986; Bosley *et al.*, 1994).

The use of incentives has been tested on selected populations in the USA, primarily the poor, and these studies have been reviewed. No clear conclusion could be drawn about the impact of financial or other incentives (Giuffrida and Torgerson, 1997). One study suggests that signing of contracts following explanation may improve medication use, but this included more complex intervention (Putnam *et al.*, 1994).

The most promising area is that of counselling and enhanced communication. A review by Stewart (1995) showed that 16 out of 21 studies found positive health improvements, suggesting that:

- a patient history that included patient perceptions/feelings, support and empathy improved symptom resolution, functional status and disease control
- discussion of management plans improved emotional state, function, symptoms and disease control.

Conducting robust randomized trials in this area is difficult, but the evidence suggests that enhanced clinician–patient communication improves health outcomes at least as much as any other intervention aimed at improving *compliance*. However, it is not clear whether improved diagnostic information gathering, decision sharing or information provision is the main factor. It seems likely, though, that whatever changes in patient information or the dispensing process are made, addressing the content and format of consultations is an important tool for improving drug use (Blenkinsopp *et al.*, 1997; Coulter *et al.*, 1999).

Conclusion

The way in which prescribed treatments are used has been perceived as a problem for many years. Since the late 1970s the research literature has contained criticism of the traditional focus on *compliance*, but remarkably little progress has been made since then. The existing literature informs us with reasonable confidence that:

- measuring *compliance* is fraught with problems
- the more objective the measure, the lower *compliance* appears to be
- techniques for collecting details of medication use from patients in the clinical setting have received little attention
- an appreciable proportion of patients do not comply, but we cannot predict which individuals these will be

- failure to comply with medication advice is associated with worse clinical outcomes
- a wide range of interventions have some effect on medication use and outcomes
- combination interventions have been shown to be most effective, but it is not clear which aspects are most important or whether a combination is required
- current methods do not identify or focus interventions on the likely cause of an individual's poor treatment use. It seems likely that such tailored interventions will be more effective than those tested to date.

We have considered the relative absence of the patient's perspective from the research literature, and can conclude that effort should be focussed on generating a greater understanding of how medication use becomes established. We have also distinguished between *compliance* and medication use, suggesting that the former should not be a goal in itself. It is clear not only that patients choose how to use their treatment, but also that they have a right to do so. In addition, the outcomes that have traditionally been defined from the medical perspective, without evidence that patients share these goals, need to be reconsidered. Unless patients' goals can be genuinely included in the prescribing process, the conflict between clinician and patient exemplified by *non-compliance* will persist. For over 20 years key authors and major reviews on medication use have been calling for a fresh approach (Sackett and Haynes, 1976; Meichenbaum and Turk, 1987; Haynes *et al.*, 1996; Marinker, 1997). Only recently has a consensus emerged that the goal of patient *compliance* with prescribed treatment regimes should be superseded by a more collaborative *concordant* approach (Blenkinsopp *et al.*, 1997). This review suggests that interventions tailored according to an understanding of a patient's *problem* promise greater success than unfocussed interventions, and reflect the shift towards more patient-centered care. It is now necessary to think through how this may be achieved. We shall expand this concept throughout the rest of the book, exploring patient behaviors in more depth and developing models for making consultations between clinicians and patients more effective in incorporating patients' preferences for medicine taking and healthcare choices.

Chapter 3

Understanding medicine taking in context

Nicky Britten

I am a reluctant pill-user, but I am beginning to be more reasonable about it. Pain-killers, I am always astonished to learn, do work. Pain is neither ennobling nor necessary. I can do without it, so I no longer fight what I used to think was a siren song of pills. I even get up at night, out of my warm but hostile bed, to take a pill because I'm finally persuaded it will take away the pain and let me sleep.

(From the journal of Regina Reibstein, who had advanced breast cancer, cited in Reibstein, 2002)

Introduction

In this chapter we shall consider medication use in its wider context. The aims of the chapter are as follows:

- to describe patients' experiences with medications
- to show that medicine taking is part of a wider context
- to help clinicians to understand medicine taking from the perspective of patients
- to demonstrate the gap between lay and professional perceptions of medicines.

The use of prescribed medicines does not occur in isolation. Rather, prescribed medicines are simply one of the many ways in which people seek to treat and manage their illnesses. An individual may be using prescribed, over-the-counter (OTC) and complementary therapies all at the same time. In order to understand this better, we shall use the well-known typology of healthcare provision described by the anthropologist Arthur Kleinman, who identified three sectors – popular, professional and folk (Kleinman, 1980). In the developed world, the popular sector includes informal healthcare carried out in the home as well as self-medication by means of over-the-counter and other remedies. The professional sector refers to orthodox medicine, and includes pharmacists and nurses as well as doctors, while the folk sector includes complementary and alternative medicine. The value of this typology is that it draws attention to the range of treatments available to people and their different (although overlapping) modalities, sources of expertise, legitimacy and availability. Thus the professional healthcare system is only part of the story. While the boundaries between these three sectors are increasingly fluid – with, for example, the increasing availability of former prescription-only medicines in supermarkets – this framework provides a useful classification. By looking at the whole range of treatments taken for all kinds of symptoms and diseases, we can better understand the context in which prescribed medicines are used. If one goal of patient-centered clinical practice is to regard the patient as a whole person, then one aim of patient-centered prescribing must be to understand the whole treatment context from the patient's perspective.

This chapter will examine sociological and anthropological studies which have revealed what people think about prescribed medicines, and how they use them. In contrast to the psychosocial models outlined in Chapter 4, these studies are mostly qualitative, and are based on interviews exploring patients' views, and also on some observational studies. There is considerable common ground with other chapters that the reader will no doubt recognize. In this chapter we take a broader perspective and consider what alternatives individuals might have, and the ways in which their context (such as their occupation, values, relatives and friends) can have an impact. The implications for communication in the consultation will be considered. Chapters 5, 6 and 7 provide many extracts from both interviews and consultations that illustrate the ideas described here.

The popular sector

The popular sector is the one in which the treatments provided by other sectors are evaluated and tested. For example, someone who has been prescribed medicines may well discuss them with friends and family both before and while taking them. This sector includes self-management of chronic diseases as well as preventive lifestyle practices such as diet and exercise regimes. It is also referred to as the family sector, as much self-care takes place within the home. However, the boundary between the popular and the professional sectors is not as clear as it sounds, because over-the-counter medicines used as part of self-management strategies can be accessed through pharmacies, and may involve discussion with a pharmacist. Given the range of treatment options available and the sometimes negative perceptions of prescribed medicines, the question arises as to how people make choices or comparisons between different kinds of treatment and different ways of responding to distress. It is sometimes said that people are too ready to 'pop pills' instead of dealing with the real social and psychological causes of their problems.

Self-care

The concept of self-care has been defined as 'action by an individual to capture or maintain a desired level of health independent of interaction with a health professional' (Clark, 2003). It includes all the ways in which people deal with their own and their families' symptoms and diseases without consulting professionals, either orthodox or not. It includes the use of traditional and home remedies, self-medication with over-the-counter treatments and medicines prescribed on earlier occasions, as well as other ways of responding to illness. The concept of illness behavior draws attention to the fact that people respond differently when they think that they are ill or when they experience something which they perceive to be a symptom.

It is often forgotten that the first choice of treatment is no treatment. Some people will automatically reach for analgesics in response to headaches or other sources of pain, while others will prefer to stop what they are doing, lie down, or even continue as before.

A significant minority of people endorse the view that most illnesses cure themselves without the need to go to the doctor (Britten *et al.*, 2002). A study in the UK found that nearly half of adults surveyed had done nothing in response to minor ailments experienced in the previous two weeks (British Market Research Bureau, 1997). Non-pharmaceutical responses to illness include changes in diet, exercise, working habits and social activities. For example, someone with stomach pains may think that they are caused by something they ate, and alter their diet, someone who is feeling depressed may try to take more exercise, or someone who is experiencing fatigue may try to work shorter hours. Although doctors may perceive that most people turn to them far too readily, it is easy to underestimate the extent of self-care, particularly if doctors rarely enquire about self-care practices. For example, one study in the UK showed that only 1 in 37 headaches experienced were reported to the family doctor (Banks *et al.*, 1975).

Traditional and home remedies

Traditional remedies and healing practices are less common in developed countries now than they were in the past, but in Canada, for example, a significant minority of Aboriginal and First Nations people still use them (Novins *et al.*, 2004). These traditional remedies are distinct from complementary and alternative medicine (CAM), which will be discussed in the section on the folk sector. The term *traditional medicine* refers to systems of healing which are embedded in historically identifiable and culturally specific beliefs about the nature of ill health that pre-date western scientific medical thinking (Thomas, 2003). These traditional treatments (e.g. acupuncture) may come under the heading of CAM if they are also used by people living in other cultures and communities, for whom such treatments are not traditional. In nineteenth-century England, people used to ask pharmacists to make up remedies according to their own recipes, but this is now an obsolete practice. Modern home remedies include the use of vinegar, Epsom salts, or lemon and garlic (not all together) for hypertension, copper wire or bracelets for arthritis, and horehound tea or buttermilk for diabetes. A study of two generations of Scottish women conducted in the late 1970s found that the older generation, who were born in the early 1920s, were more likely than the younger generation to talk about home remedies (Blaxter and Paterson, 1982). Data from the USA suggest that home remedies such as steam inhalation are used to treat respiratory problems, including colds, coughs and sore throats. A survey conducted in North-West England in the 1990s found that over a quarter of people who reported one or more days of restricted activity due to their health, illness or injury had taken home remedies (Hassell *et al.*, 1998). Studies of Afro-Caribbean groups in the UK have shown that the use of traditional herbal and home remedies is fairly common, both in place of and alongside prescribed medicines. Patients who are being treated with drugs for hypertension may still use traditional West Indian herbal remedies, either at the same time or while taking 'drug holidays' (Morgan and Watkins, 1988).

Interestingly, like many forms of treatment, home remedies appear to be viewed as safer than and in many cases preferable to prescribed drugs. A study of hypothetical choices in the USA, which compared preferences for a high-risk drug, a low-risk drug and a home remedy for the treatment of sore throat, hypertension, arthritis or gastro-enteritis, showed that 72% of respondents chose the home remedy. These remedies were a salt-water gargle for sore throat, low-salt diet for hypertension, a heat pad for arthritis, and a clear liquid diet for gastroenteritis. Those who chose the home remedies had concerns about the potential side-effects of the drug remedies (Povar *et al.*, 1984). Although the results of a hypothetical study do not necessarily tell us about actual behavior, they suggest that prescribers could usefully explore the use of home remedies with their patients.

Overall, however, little is known about the use of home and traditional remedies, as they have not been the subject of much research. It is very likely that these traditional remedies are regarded as 'natural', and that when people speak of natural remedies, it is these kinds of home and traditional remedies to which they are referring.

Self-medication

The popular sector also includes self-medication with over-the-counter pharmaceuticals. Some over-the-counter preparations may be based on traditional remedies such as honey and lemon, with the inclusion of some analgesic. Others are milder versions of prescription drugs, or may be drugs that were formerly prescription only. One of the reasons for the deregulation of prescription medicines is to encourage people to take responsibility for their own healthcare, as well as transferring costs from the health service budget to individual patients. A survey in the UK showed that, in response to minor ailments in the previous two weeks, over a quarter of adults had used an over-the-counter medicine, while 14% had used a prescription medicine that was already in the house (British Market Research Bureau, 1997). The common types of problems for which people treat themselves include headache, athlete's foot, dandruff, heartburn, migraine, vaginal yeast infections and period pains. Some of these problems may be long term and hence also treated with prescribed drugs, leading to a risk of multiple treatments and consequent interactions or overdose. The evidence suggests that doctors do not ask patients about the use of over-the-counter treatments, and that patients do not tell them about it (Stevenson *et al.*, 2003). On the whole, people tend to regard over-the-counter treatments as safer than prescribed medicines, believing that if they were not safe, they would not be so widely available. They may be unaware of the dangers of interactions between over-the-counter and prescribed medicines, or of the fact that the ingredients may be the same. Someone who is taking an over-the-counter and a prescribed analgesic may not realize that both often include acetaminophen (paracetamol).

Thus within the popular sector people adopt a wide range of self-care practices that clinicians may want to enquire about. This environment forms the backdrop against which any suggested prescribed treatment will be judged. Strong views in favour of home remedies or against drugs will influence decisions about their use. This may include a family or traditional folklore based on collective experiences, and any diagnosis or prescription that contradicts these beliefs will not be readily accepted.

The professional sector

In most countries, prescribed medicines can only be obtained from licensed doctors, nurses and pharmacists. These professional groups thus control access to medicines, determining the types of medicine, the doses and the quantities in which they are supplied. Thus from the layperson's point of view, medicines and healthcare professionals are intimately connected. The use of the same word 'medicine' to denote both the profession and the treatment underlines this close relationship. Healthcare professionals' knowledge of therapeutics is gained through many years of training and experience, which may make it difficult for them to appreciate that others might have their own experiential knowledge and a different belief system. Although lay knowledge may well be informed by professional knowledge, the two are by no means synonymous. Even the terminology can lead to misunderstandings. For example, it is clear that lay understanding of the terms *addiction* and *dependence* extends far beyond the pharmacological meanings of these terms. People express fears about becoming addicted to antibiotics, and to drugs for epilepsy, hypertension and rheumatism, as well as to tranquillizers and other psychotropic medicines. For some people, the terms 'medicine' and 'drug' are interchangeable, while for others the term 'drug' has only negative connotations. This suggests that in any discussion about medicines, apparently obvious terms may need to be clarified.

Attitudes towards medicines

Studies of lay beliefs about medicines have shown that people have a range of positive and negative views that recur across different populations, disease groups and countries. People say less about their positive views, perhaps because these represent a perspective that is taken for granted, and dominant, about the necessity, effectiveness and safety of prescribed medicines. In a questionnaire study conducted in south London, the majority of respondents agreed that modern medicines have improved people's health and that medicines aid recovery from illness (Britten *et al.*, 2002). For many people, taking medicines is not problematic if they trust the clinician and are willing to do as he or she recommends.

However, there is a range of commonly expressed negative attitudes about prescribed medicines. Some of these represent non-specific dislike of medicines and medicine taking expressed by people both with and without chronic conditions that require long-term medication. Clearly, for some people, dislike of medicine taking is closely bound up with a dislike of being ill. Over 86% of respondents in one study agreed with the statement 'I prefer not to take any medicine if I can avoid it' (Britten *et al.*, 2002). Interestingly, another study of people visiting their family doctor found that most of the respondents expressed this kind of aversion when being interviewed by the researcher at home beforehand, but did not say anything to their doctor (Britten *et al.*, 2004). Although much of the evidence about aversion to medicines comes from studies of attitudes to psychotropic medicines, such attitudes are also expressed about all other kinds of medicine. For example, one study found that more than 80% of a sample of people attending a rheumatology clinic spontaneously expressed dislike of having to take drugs at all (Donovan and Blake, 1992). Fears about dependency and addiction are widespread, and cannot be assessed easily. These fears refer to addiction and psychological dependency, as well as concerns about tolerance. People may take 'drug holidays' if they are worried that their medicines will cease to be effective if taken over a long period of time (Urquhart, 2005). Such concerns are not necessarily related to the known pharmacological properties of the medicines concerned, and point to the need for communication and accurate information to inform people's decision-making processes. Other concerns which affect medicine taking include the fear that symptoms of other diseases may be masked in the process.

A more specific theme is the view that manufactured medicines are unnatural. This perceived 'unnaturalness' has been expressed in relation to oral contraception, benzodiazepines, childhood vaccinations, antidepressants, antihypertensive medication and many other medicines. This concept of unnaturalness is closely linked to that of harm and, conversely, substances that are perceived as natural are often also perceived as safe. Unnatural chemicals may also be contrasted with natural experiences such as the menopause, contributing to some women's preference not to take hormone replacement therapy, even before more recent safety concerns emerged (Hunter *et al.*, 1997). However, the meaning of the word 'natural' is far from self-evident, and is not always made clear in the literature. In some studies, natural substances are those which are made from plants or herbs. In a Swedish study on natural medicines, several categories of meaning were identified (Fallsberg, 1991). Natural products were those made from plants but also those whose naturalness was preserved during processing. A natural product had to be processed as little as possible and the genuine substance had to be kept as intact as possible. Another category of natural product consisted of substances either originating in or needed by the human body. They could also be defined as intrinsically weak, so that because of their low concentration they were either non-toxic or less toxic than drugs. However, the distinction between natural and unnatural medicines is not clear-cut, as some people recognize that natural medicines may also be manufactured and they are not always regarded as safe.

Clearly, if people have these ambivalent ideas about medicines, the question arises as to how this affects their medicine taking. Chapter 2 established that up to half of prescribed medication is not taken as directed. This finding applies to most disease areas, population groups and geographical locations. Qualitative research helps us to understand people's attitudes to medicines and the ways in which people actually use their medicines.

Testing medicines

A recent synthesis of 10 years of qualitative literature about lay perspectives on medicines found considerable evidence about the ways in which patients test their medicines, although few studies explicitly addressed this (Pound *et al.*, 2005). The studies that were included in the synthesis were concerned with drugs for a range of conditions, including HIV/AIDS, hypertension, diabetes, digestive disorders, rheumatoid arthritis, mental illness and asthma. A range of different approaches to testing medicines were noted. The commonest approach was to try out a medicine and weigh up the costs and benefits – a rational balancing act. Other methods included discontinuing the medicine and seeing what happened as a pragmatic assessment, and observing others. Although people took their medicines for a variety of reasons, and not only to obtain symptom relief or cure, they also described a great many negative effects that mitigated against medicine taking. These included not only a range of side-effects, which were particularly varied and unpleasant in the case of medicines for schizophrenia and HIV/AIDS, but also effects on people's social, family and working lives. For some individuals, the side-effects of the medicines and the damage to their social lives were such that they were not prepared to continue taking the medicines. Thus the pragmatic evaluation could inform a considered decision. The unpleasant effects could also persuade people that the drugs were doing them more harm than good and lead to a more emotive response. These findings accord with Leventhal's cycles of appraisal described in Chapter 4. Treatment for HIV/AIDS could be experienced as more threatening to patients' well-being than the disease itself. As well as weighing up the costs and benefits, people also tried stopping their medication to see what happened. If they felt worse as a result, then they were more likely to resume their medication. If they felt no different or even better after quitting their medication, they had less incentive to resume it.

People employed other methods of testing their medicines, including the use of objective and subjective indicators, and observing others. In a condition such as hypertension, there are few subjective indicators to help people to monitor the effectiveness of treatment, so they are more reliant on objective measurements taken by health professionals. In the case of HIV, people are able to use both subjective and objective indicators of the progress of disease, and when these conflict, subjective indicators may have more influence on the use of medicines than objective indicators. This suggests that in other conditions where both subjective and objective indicators are available, objective tests may be less persuasive than health professionals realize. A study of women taking AZT found that they were often more influenced by their observation of how others were responding to treatment than by their doctors' advice. If their own observations convinced them that people on treatment did less well than those who were not being treated, they would decide not to take treatment themselves (Siegel and Gorey, 1997). This suggests that clinicians should involve patients in the process of monitoring their progress.

One of the difficulties that people experience when testing their medicines is knowing which effects are due to the medicine and which are due to the disease. If symptoms of the disease are attributed to the treatment, people may quit their medicines as a result. There is clearly an important role here for health professionals in helping patients to assess which effects are due to which causes. Of course this requires that the whole question of effects and side-effects is discussed openly. In one study, doctors substituted patients' usual brand of proton pump inhibitor for a cheaper brand, and reduced the dose at the same time. This made it very difficult for patients to test the efficacy of the new drug, as they had not been told about the reduced dose (Pollock and Grime, 2000). If patients are not given adequate information about their medicines, it is very difficult for them to assess them appropriately, and they may make poor decisions as a result.

Medicine taking has an impact on people's identity, and labels them as having a particular disease. This is particularly problematic with stigmatized diseases such as HIV/AIDS and mental illness, but also with diseases like asthma. People with asthma who do not accept the diagnosis are unlikely to take preventive treatments, and may rely solely on symptomatic medication (Adams *et al.*, 1997). Taking medicine is a reminder of illness, so that the act of taking tablets can threaten people's sense of normality. Taking medication in front of other people can jeopardize social status. For example, those who have not disclosed their disease to employers may feel embarrassed or stigmatized by taking medicines in the workplace.

Taking medicines

Even if a decision has been made to take the medicine as prescribed, factors such as the ability to pay or repeat-prescribing arrangements may make this difficult. Interruptions to daily routine, being away from home, forgetfulness or feeling stressed can all interfere with medicine taking.

People take different approaches to their medicines and offer different accounts when asked. They may accept their medicines either actively or passively, they may reject medication or they may modify their regimen (Pound *et al.*, 2005). Most research has focussed on those who modify their regimens, as those who accept their medication are not considered to be a problem, and those who have rejected their medicines may also reject the invitation to participate in research and may be difficult to trace. Very little longitudinal research has been carried out on this topic, so we do not know the extent to which people's views and behaviors change with time. It seems very likely that views about medicines are context specific, and that someone who has rejected the treatment of a minor complaint may then accept treatment for a life-threatening condition. However, the quote from Regina Reibstein's journal cited above shows that, even while dying in great pain, anti-drug attitudes can remain powerful.

People who have accepted medicine taking without necessarily giving it a great deal of thought may be characterized as passive accepters (Pound *et al.*, 2005). They may well have relinquished control of their illness to their doctors, and when asked, may say that they trust their doctors and will do whatever their doctors recommend. The lack of reflection associated with passive acceptance means that, when interviewed, they may not have very much to say. Their stories may illustrate occasions when their normal routine which is taken for granted is disrupted. By contrast, active accepters are people who have thought about taking their medicines, and may have tested them, and who take them as prescribed. Pound refers to this group as showing 'purposeful adherence.' They may have concerns and worries, or they may not, but in either case they have made a conscious decision to pursue the prescribed regimen.

Other people may reject their medicines, either after a period of testing or not. These rejecters or sceptics may prefer to remain in control by using alternative therapies or by tolerating their symptoms (Pound *et al.*, 2005). This group is likely to include people who are critical of both modern medicine and doctors, and who describe pharmaceuticals as damaging and unnatural. They may be more likely to use CAM.

The group about whom most is known consists of those who modify their prescribed regimens. Studies of people taking medicines for a range of conditions, including rheumatoid arthritis, hypertension, HIV, epilepsy and asthma, have shown that self-regulation is common. This may result from a process of testing, and balancing the costs and benefits of taking medicines. This modification may also give people a sense of being in control of their disease and its treatment, rather than being controlled.

People use a variety of methods for modifying their regimen (Pound *et al.*, 2005). A common strategy is to minimize medicine intake, and indeed the stronger the drug, the greater is the desire to reduce the dose. People even try to minimize their consumption of drugs such as proton pump inhibitors and benzodiazepines, which professionals also think are overused. Other strategies, which also have the effect of reducing consumption, include using medicines symptomatically rather than regularly. Even in conditions such as hypertension, which is regarded by professionals as an asymptomatic condition, some people will take their medicines when they feel the need to, and not otherwise. The same has been found for rheumatoid arthritis and bipolar depression.

People also modify their medication regimens in relation to their social activities, particularly alcohol consumption. Fears about potential interactions between prescribed medicines and alcohol can lead people to stay off their medicines when partying. This may account for the observation that 'drug holidays' occur more often at weekends.

Those who are taking proton pump inhibitors may adjust their medication as necessary on the basis of what they have eaten or are about to eat. Another strategy of self-regulation is informed by the desire to decrease adverse effects. People may reduce or skip doses in order to reduce adverse effects, sometimes waiting until these effects have passed before starting to take their medicines again. Those on multiple medication may decide to take medicines separately to prevent them from interacting with each other. Those who are concerned about the build-up of toxicity in their bodies may take drug holidays in order to cleanse their systems. Drug holidays may consist of a short or long period of abstinence, or they can take the form of a regular drug-free day once a week. People may also modify their medication to fit in with their daily lives, including work and family life.

Managing everyday life

For many people who are struggling to cope with chronic disease, the ability to live a normal life and meet their social obligations is more important to them than symptom control. Prescribed medicines may help people to meet their various obligations but at the same time serve as evidence of an inability to perform such roles. The demands of family life and paid employment are the highest priority for many people, and medicine use may be tailored to these competing demands. Studies of the use of tranquillizers have shown how these medicines help people to maintain their roles as wives, mothers, homemakers and employees (Cooperstock and Lennard, 1979). For those who are unable to change their work situation, taking tranquillizers could be the only way of alleviating sometimes incapacitating symptoms and allowing them to retain their paid employment. Similarly, those who are taking antiretroviral treatment may alter their regimen to fit in with their daily schedule, so that they can continue their life without too much disruption. Some may feel that strict adherence is neither attainable nor realistic.

Thus the management of adverse effects is one of the reasons why people self-regulate their medicines. On the whole, patients want to have more information about their medicines than they receive, and this may help them to appraise treatment more accurately. The issue of unavoidable side-effects is difficult, and is one of the reasons why some people turn to complementary and alternative therapies.

Clinicians need to understand their patients' priorities, as well as their experiences of side-effects, if they want to know how prescribed treatments are actually being used (or not). Instead of thinking about medicine taking in terms of compliance, they could see their role as supporting patients' problem-solving and self-management strategies.

The folk sector

Types of complementary and alternative treatment

This sector consists of various different forms of *complementary and alternative medicine (CAM)*. The latter is now established as a generic term to embrace both of these types of healing systems. They may be defined as those forms of healing that are not usually taught in medical schools, or are not part of the politically dominant healthcare system, although both of these aspects are changing. Thomas (2003) has classified the various types of CAM therapy under five headings:

- ethnic medical systems, such as traditional Chinese medicine
- non-allopathic systems, such as homeopathy
- manual therapies, such as osteopathy
- mind–body therapies, such as Reiki
- nature cure therapies, such as naturopathy.

There are some common threads to their various different modes of action, namely the support of self-healing processes, an individualized approach to diagnosis and treatment, and working with rather than against symptoms to uncover the underlying causes of ill health.

Estimates of the numbers of people who consult CAM practitioners depend on the definitions used, but suggest that there are significant levels of use in Australia, the USA, Canada and the UK. Studies conducted in the UK and the USA suggest that between a quarter and half of the people in these countries have consulted a complementary practitioner at some time in their life (Thomas, 2003). Estimates for visits in the previous year vary from 13% to 20% in the last year, which rises to 30–40% if over-the-counter CAM products are included. By 1997, the number of visits to complementary practitioners in the USA had probably exceeded those to primary care physicians. In the UK, some complementary therapy is available free of charge within the National Health Service, but provision is dependent on the prevailing policy and funding climate. In most countries, CAM represents a form of private healthcare, and access to care depends on the ability to pay.

Users of CAM therapies tend to be younger and better educated than non-users. Women and non-manual workers also tend to use CAM more often than men and manual workers. However, users of CAM are very far from being a homogenous group, and the socioeconomic status of users varies between therapies. Musculoskeletal problems are the dominant clinical reason for consulting CAM practitioners in Canada, Australia, the UK and the USA (Thomas, 2003). Other presenting problems include psychological problems, fatigue, and respiratory and digestive problems. Some of these problems are of long standing, and surveys suggest a mean duration of 8 to 9 years. People who consult chiropractors are less likely to have chronic problems, as are children.

Thomas (2003) has identified a range of reasons for seeking CAM care, some of which are 'pull factors' to do with the attractions of CAM care, while others are 'push factors' that reflect problems with orthodox care and attitudes to science. It is the latter which have more implications for prescribers and for the conducting of orthodox consultations.

'Pull factors'

The 'pull factors' include lifestyle choice, active well-being and health maintenance, and pragmatism and anticipated symptom relief. The first of these refers to the compatibility between users' values and beliefs and the principles underlying most CAM therapies. Those with a holistic philosophy of health are more likely to choose CAM therapies than those who do not espouse such a philosophy. Specific beliefs which motivate people to use CAM include the belief that CAM has the ability to enhance the immune system (Boon *et al.*, 1999). Some people use CAM therapies to maintain their health and as a preventive strategy, and may seek treatment even though they have no current health problems. Thus CAM therapies, including bodywork therapies such as massage, and osteopathy, can help people to take responsibility for their health. Those without a philosophical commitment to holistic care may consult CAM practitioners in the hope of obtaining symptom relief. The range of perceived benefits is similarly broad. For some people, their main goal is reduced dependence on long-term treatments for chronic conditions, or the amelioration of side-effects, rather than symptom reduction. People may also choose to consult CAM practitioners because they perceive them to be better listeners and to provide more emotional support than conventional practitioners (Boon *et al.*, 2000).

'Push factors'

The 'push factors' include dissatisfaction with orthodox care, and the search for a satisfactory therapeutic relationship. Dissatisfaction with orthodox care has four elements:

- ineffectiveness of orthodox care
- poor communication with doctors
- a perceived lack of control or choice in conventional care
- the perceived dangers and side-effects of some orthodox treatments.

Criticisms of doctors' communication may be voiced by those with undiagnosed conditions who feel that their problems are not being taken seriously, but may also be expressed by those who feel that doctors are over-reliant on prescription drugs and unwilling to explore other ways of treating disease. Some patients are resentful of doctors who reach for the prescription pad as a way of terminating the consultation, and would prefer discussion of self-management, including diet and exercise. Given the fact that CAM users tend to be younger and more highly educated, it might be expected that they wish to feel in control of their healthcare. As already noted, there is widespread ambivalence about prescribed medicines and concern about side-effects, which motivates some people to seek alternative methods of treatment. Asthma sufferers, in choosing acupuncture treatment, may have as their main aim the avoidance or reduction of steroid drugs (Paterson and Britten, 1999). A study of men with prostate cancer found that some had chosen to use CAM because they viewed conventional medical treatments as having significant adverse effects, including impotence and incontinence (Boon *et al.*, 2003). People may feel that doctors and orthodox medicine cannot help them much if the treatments that have been offered have been of limited benefit. Some people may feel rejected by orthodox medicine. Others may feel that although orthodox treatment works for them, it is unacceptable, possibly due to its side-effects. Those who are seeking a satisfactory therapeutic relationship may value the quality of listening, holistic care and the philosophy of partnership that characterize CAM care. Although these characteristics are not exclusive to CAM practitioners, or even exhibited by all of them, they represent an ethos that is widely known. While orthodox practitioners may attribute the appeal of CAM treatment to the longer consultation times, time alone is no guarantee of a holistic approach or a respectful attitude.

Thus doctors' use of prescription writing as a way of reducing consultation times may have the unintended consequence of motivating some patients to seek other forms of healthcare.

Supplement or substitute?

People consult CAM therapists about a range of chronic problems, choose different therapies for different problems, and may continue their treatment as a preventive measure. Most of these people will have consulted their orthodox doctors about their problem, and may still be receiving orthodox treatment. Some will be attending other CAM therapists, and many will be continuing self-help measures. The use of CAM treatments is as much a supplement to orthodox treatment as it is a substitute for it, which suggests that CAM and orthodox practitioners need to understand one another's approaches. CAM therapists are often asked by their clients to explain the nature of their biomedical diagnoses and treatments, and to help them to make treatment choices.

Communication in the consultation and implications for prescribers

It is clear that the context in which prescribed medicines are taken is broad, and that people use a much wider range of treatments than are discussed in most consultations. There is widespread ambivalence about prescribed medicines, coupled with the perception that over-the-counter medicines and complementary treatments are usually harmless. In this concluding section we shall discuss the implications of these considerations for prescribers. The issues for prescribers are twofold – first, the variable quality and quantity of communication about prescribed medicines, and secondly, the paucity of communication about over-the-counter and CAM treatments.

Communication about prescribed treatments

A recent review of the literature on two-way communication about medicines found little evidence of shared decision making, and concluded that clinicians can act as either facilitators or barriers in terms of communicating with patients about their medicines (Cox *et al.*, 2004). Many patients do want to discuss their medicines with doctors, especially with regard to side-effects. As already discussed, people have concerns about their medicines, but do not often get the opportunity to discuss them with their doctors. Patients are more likely to express a concern if their doctors explicitly ask them about their medicines, if they rate their health as poor, if they consult with younger rather than older doctors, and if they are using more medications. Consultation recordings show that doctors may not even name a drug that is being prescribed for the first time. When patients do ask questions about their medicines, they do not always even get a response, let alone an answer. The benefits of prescribed medicines are discussed more often than the dangers, even though patients want to know about side-effects and have access to other sources of information about them. Patients may not trust a doctor who only talks about the benefits of treatment without acknowledging the potential problems. Doctors do not usually involve patients in choosing treatments. However a study which examined the effects of patient participation in discussions about medicines showed that greater patient involvement was associated with greater subsequent understanding of the treatment, more satisfaction with the visit and their doctor's behavior, and less regret about the treatment decision (Siminoff *et al.*, 2000).

Research studies suggest that roughly half of patients on long-term medication ask doctors questions about their medicines (Cox *et al.*, 2004). The commonest questions asked by patients concern which medicines they are taking, quantity and supply, the conditions that the medicines are for, the dosage, purpose and interval, the name of the medicine, and barriers and side-effects. These questions can be put more succinctly as follows. What is it? Is it necessary? What is it for? Does it work? Is it safe? Clinicians should check with their patients to see whether they have unanswered questions in these or other areas related to their medicines. The reasons that patients give for not asking more questions include the perception that doctors are too busy, and a lack of awareness of what questions they could ask.

When consulting family doctors, patients have complex agendas with regard to many aspects of their illness experience. One UK study found that voiced agenda items included symptoms, requests for diagnoses and prescriptions (Barry *et al.*, 2000). Unvoiced agenda items included worries about the possible diagnosis and what the future held, patients' own ideas about what was wrong with them, side-effects, not wanting a prescription, and information about their social context. Unvoiced agenda items often led to poor outcomes, including unwanted prescriptions, non-use of prescriptions and non-adherence to treatment. The same study identified 14 categories of misunderstanding between patients and doctors which had potential or actual adverse consequences for taking medicines (Britten *et al.*, 2000). All of the misunderstandings were associated with lack of patient participation in the consultation. Patients did not voice their expectations and preferences, or they did not voice their responses to doctors' decisions and actions. Misunderstandings arose due to lack of exchange of relevant information in both directions, as a result of conflicting information or attributions, when the patient failed to understand the doctor's diagnostic or treatment decision, and from actions taken to preserve the doctor–patient relationship. For example, a doctor might think that the parent of a small child expects an antibiotic, and prescribe one in order to maintain the patient–doctor relationship. The parent might have preferred not to give the child an antibiotic, but felt that one was necessary by virtue of the fact that the doctor had prescribed one. In this way a patient may take a medicine that is thought to be unnecessary by the doctor out of fear that further treatment may be withheld.

The kinds of misunderstandings that were identified in this study were based on inaccurate assumptions and guesses by both parties. Doctors either thought that they already knew the patients' preferences, or they considered that such knowledge was unimportant. In particular, doctors seemed to be unaware of the relevance of patients' ideas for successful prescribing, and of the fairly widespread aversion to taking medicines (Britten *et al.*, 2004). Although patients expressed aversion in the research interviews, few did so in the consultations, and when they did, some did so indirectly or as asides. Other patients expressed aversion directly, but even in these cases there was no further discussion of the patients' views. Whether patients expressed their aversion or not, and whether they expressed it directly or indirectly, doctors did not discuss the patients' views of medicines with them. The implications of this study are that clinicians need to enquire about patients' views of medicines when they are considering writing a prescription as well as when they are not. When patients say that they do not want to take medicines, clinicians could usefully explore their reasons, and discuss the benefits as well as the risks of such action. In both cases, consideration should be given to alternative treatments, including no treatment. Clinicians would be well advised to pay attention to patients' expression of aversion to medicines in the form of conversational asides, because the information conveyed indirectly may still be relevant and even crucial for the later taking of medicines.

Communication about non-prescribed treatments

In relation to over-the-counter and CAM treatments, patients' willingness to reveal their use of non-prescribed treatments is influenced by their source and by the perceived legitimacy of the treatment. Treatments that are prescribed or recommended by doctors may be perceived by patients as having greater legitimacy than those provided by pharmacists or CAM practitioners (Stevenson *et al.*, 2002). If doctors endorse or recommend treatments that are available over the counter or provided by CAM therapists, patients are more likely to admit to using such treatments. However, many doctors do not ask patients about their use of non-prescribed treatments (either over the counter or CAM). This may be due to their own lack of knowledge about these treatments, or to the fact that they do not regard them as important. However, patients may interpret the absence of enquiry into their use of other treatments as an indication that doctors disapprove of them. Certainly if patients have felt criticized for their use of other treatments in the past, they are less likely to volunteer this information again. A qualitative study of breast cancer survivors in Canada who were using CAM reported that either their physicians did not want to know about the alternative therapies they were taking, or they responded with scepticism to all CAM (Boon *et al.*, 1999). A quantitative follow-up study by the same authors found that less than half of the women who were using some form of CAM said that their physicians knew that they were taking CAM (Boon *et al.*, 2000).

Conclusion

If clinicians want to understand the whole treatment context, they need to find out about the range of treatments that their patients are using, and let their patients know that discussion of over-the-counter and CAM treatments is legitimate. The move to more open communication and shared decision making means that clinicians need to discuss all of the ways in which patients have attempted to deal with their symptoms, and to accept that people do use a wide range of treatments. Professionals need to appreciate the relevance and importance of engaging with patients' perspectives. Research in this area has shown that few practitioners actively engage with patients' perspectives on their treatment regimes, presumably because they do not see the value of doing so. It seems likely, given the extent of *discrepant* medication use with prescribed treatments and the range of other treatments used by many patients, that most prescribers have little idea about the totality of treatments used by their patients, or the ways in which prescribed treatments are used. Clinicians may be tempted to think that non-compliance is an issue for the patients of other practitioners, but not their own. Even if they appreciate that this is a problem for their own patients, they may not have accepted the significance of the patients' own ideas and beliefs in determining their medicine-taking behavior. As patients are often inhibited during the consultation, prescribers need to make an effort to find out what they are doing if they are to understand the social, psychological and even pharmacological context within which their treatments are prescribed. Questions that practitioners could ask include what other ways patients have used to treat themselves, whether these have helped, how patients feel about the treatments prescribed for them, and whether they have any problems with them. If clinicians find out about the ways in which patients have tested their prescribed medicines, they will understand better the criteria that patients are using and the outcomes that they are hoping for. If clinicians explicitly mention the potential side-effects, this will produce a more balanced discussion than one which only focuses on the potential benefits. Clinicians may then be in a position to help patients to distinguish between the side-effects of medicines and the symptoms of the condition for which they are being prescribed.

Patients' use of over-the-counter and CAM therapies, or even their use of prescribed medicines, may be suboptimal or even dangerous from a professional perspective. Prescribed medicines may be taken in sub-therapeutic doses. Over-the-counter medicines may have potential interactions with prescribed ones. CAM therapists may provide treatments that healthcare professionals regard as ineffective. The evidence so far suggests that many doctors do not enquire about the use of over-the-counter and CAM therapies, and that there is little discussion of other forms of treatment. If doctors discover that patients have been using treatments which they consider to be unsafe or ineffective, they need to be careful not to criticize these choices while explaining the risks attached to them. Patients who feel that their actions or choices have been criticized, especially if the reasons for these choices have not been explored, may be less likely to admit to them on other occasions.

In aiming for patient-centered prescribing, clinicians need to recognize the importance of patients' ideas and values in influencing their medicine taking. Failure to appreciate this can lead to ineffective communication and consequent problems with medicine use.

Chapter 4

Understanding medicine taking: models and explanations

Brian Williams

Introduction

Chapters 2 and 3 argue that prescribers must have a degree of insight into their patients' perspectives before patient-centered prescribing and a more concordant relationship can result (Weston and Brown, 1995). These perspectives include both the patient's beliefs about and experience of their illness (the subjective experience and interpretation of disease) (Eisenberg, 1977), and their views about the way in which healthcare interventions are impacting or likely to impact on their everyday life (Williams and Grant, 1998). Gaining an insight into these issues is challenging. It requires both the will to enquire *and* the ability to access what is often a set of hidden or ill-defined beliefs and experiences. This chapter provides an overview of academic and empirical research that sheds light on these issues. Some readers may already be familiar with some of this research and the key issues to which it relates. Others may feel that an overview of applied, but still academic, research is less relevant than the actual 'how to' of patient-centered prescribing. Both groups may wish to skip this chapter and turn straight to Chapter 5. They can return to this chapter at a later stage when or if curiosity about the theoretical underpinnings and evidence base of the models presented in Section 2 arises.

Recent years have seen an increase in the number of communication skills training courses available for clinicians, and the publication of a number of studies which suggest that doctors' attitudes towards using a patient-centered approach are more favourable. For example, a recent survey of 64 family doctors and 410 of their patients in the UK found that practitioners believed that instead of focussing simply on the patient's clinical problem, it was important to acknowledge their feelings and avoid medical jargon. In fact doctors rated receptiveness and the affective content of the relationship as even more important for a good consultation than many patients did (Ogden *et al.*, 2002).

Although doctors are increasingly willing to access patients' views, many still overestimate just how patient-centered their consultations tend to be and underestimate the degree to which they (the doctors) direct the conversation. In a study of 271 consultations, Makoul *et al.* (1995) found that doctors believed that they had discussed a patient's ability to follow instructions in 49% of cases, whereas it only actually occurred in 8%. In terms of discussion that was initiated by doctors in the consultation,

87% related to instructions for medication use, 54% related to intended benefits, 22% related to possible side-effects, 15% related to patients' opinions about the medication, and 5% related to patients' ability to follow the treatment plan (Makoul *et al.*, 1995). Such discrepancies are concerning, as they clearly indicate a tendency for some doctors to be overly directive. As Chapter 1 made clear, being patient-centered involves more than simply providing information and letting the patient decide. It includes discussing the patient's perspective on their illness, the way in which it has impacted on their life, and any hopes, goals, fears or concerns with regard to treatment.

While a favorable attitude towards patient-centered care, and prescribing in particular, is desirable, it is not enough. Since patient-centered prescribing is predicated on the importance of patients' beliefs, hopes and goals, the clinician also requires the technical and interpersonal skills necessary to discover what these are. Most clinicians would quite rightly regard attempting to accurately uncover their patients' beliefs and experiences, let alone their medication behaviors, as far from easy. And yet this is what is required for prescribing to become truly patient-centered. While it may not be easy to access a patient's beliefs and experiences, particularly within a time-limited consultation, the clinician need not commence this process with an entirely blank mind. With a knowledge of symptom patterns and familiar disease presentations derived from formal training and years of clinical experience, diagnosis can often be determined very quickly. Forms of 'pattern recognition' are developed. Similarly, a prior knowledge of what attitudes, beliefs, practices, fears and concerns are common among particular patient groups can help to improve both the effectiveness and the efficiency of a consultation which is aiming to achieve a level of shared understanding. A clinician who understands why people tend to react as they do will find it far easier to recognize and predict behaviors. An open mind may well be helpful – a blank one will frustrate everyone.

The purpose of this chapter is therefore to provide a knowledge base that clinicians can draw upon to help them to elicit and interpret their patients' beliefs, concerns and practices more effectively. Although the specific skills are considered in Chapter 6, it is necessary to have a framework in place to help to understand the responses that patients may give. Just as clinical history taking is inefficient and often fruitless without an appreciation of the potential disease processes, so too attempts to understand behavior may be improved through knowledge of the underlying theory. We shall begin by briefly reviewing the obstacles that make it difficult to access or even recognize the patient's perspective as a legitimate or fruitful avenue of enquiry. Next we shall examine some of the models that have been developed in response to the need to understand patient behavior more fully. A brief critique is then provided in an attempt to put these psychosocial models in context and highlight their limitations. The aim is to focus on models that are thought to relate to medication-related behaviors and to see how these can help, rather than to provide an overview of all the behavioral models or concepts.

Obstacles to understanding medicine taking

In order to truly hear what a patient says, a clinician must be aware of and guard against assumptions, tendencies or prejudices that might influence both their willingness to inquire about their patients' views and their subsequent interpretation of the responses. Prior to the evolution of patient-centered care and the move from *compliance/*

adherence to concordance, patients who acted contrary to medical recommendations were commonly regarded as either behaving irrationally or failing to comprehend what they had been told. The assumption that underlay this view was that people would and should act in logical and reasonable ways once they had been adequately informed of their circumstances. However, this view assumes that the clinician and the patient both agree that the '(bio)medical model' is the definitive and correct approach to disease, and that the patient should be largely deferent towards the doctor, since he or she has unique access to this approach.

It can be argued that the traditional 'medical model', which has been the focus of so much criticism, was really an artificial construct from a predominantly academic debate – a straw man that did not really exist in its much caricatured form. At the centre of this model was, and is, a conceptualization of the body as a complex machine, and a corresponding notion of normal or proper functioning (Engel, 1977, 1980). The history of modern medicine is a history of discovery of the human body, taking it apart, identifying the function of individual organs or components and exploring their interrelationships. Health is considered to be a state in which the body is functioning properly, whereas illness reflects a deviation from normality. The role of the doctor is to mend the machine and return it to correct functioning (i.e. return it to 'health'). The belief that someone who is ill will seek help and follow a course of action recommended by a physician rests on the assumption that they accept the medical model as the authoritative explanation of health and disease. We know that this assumption was always highly questionable, and recent challenges to it are forcing changes in the practice of medicine. Rather than adopting the wholesale allopathic models of health and disease, we now know that a range of lay models of anatomy and physiology and definitions of both illness and health exist both within and across cultures. These include humoral theories, 'plumbing' models (Kleinman *et al.*, 1978) and symbolic anatomies (Helman, 1998), while definitions of health go beyond the absence of disease to include functionality, energy/vitality and contentedness (Blaxter, 1983, 1990). Importantly, these are not simply to be found in exotic locations around the globe, but in all societies, irrespective of any institutional acceptance of western medicine.

Given the existence of these alternative understandings of the human body, it is possible for people to behave in ways that may appear to be irrational but which are in fact quite consistent with their own lay understandings and models. Rather than giving in to an assumption of irrationality on behalf of the patient, we would argue that it is better to assume the existence of an underlying rationale and discover misunderstanding and confusion (if they exist) in the process of trying to comprehend what that rationale *is*. Such an approach recognizes the need for and benefit of identifying a patient's *own* concerns and beliefs in achieving a patient-centered outcome and as a method of achieving behavioral change where that is appropriate (Rollnick *et al.*, 1999).

Another factor that may sometimes prove to be an obstacle to understanding patients' medication use relates to the perceived roles of both the doctor and the patient. Roles can be defined as bundles of expectations, rights and responsibilities. These may lead patients to believe that it is inappropriate to raise particular issues with a clinician and, likewise, the clinician may regard certain lines of enquiry as being outside his or her sphere of responsibility. For example, during a conference discussion in Sydney in 1998 on the role of quality-of-life measures in evaluating patient-centered services, one researcher indicated that although he worked in a mental health clinic, he preferred to use generic quality-of-life measures rather than one that only measured dimensions of mental health or well-being. He had found that many patients failed to report physical problems such as pain, as they did not regard it as the service's role to address these kinds of problems. The generic quality-of-life tool picked up these unreported physical complaints. A study by Williams has shown how these perceptions of the role of services (and its constituent parts) can lead to high levels of reported satisfaction despite poor aspects of healthcare experiences (Williams *et al.*, 1998). Role perceptions can therefore obstruct the development of a range of patient-centered activities, including prescribing.

Understanding illness behavior

The history and breadth of the social and behavioral sciences demonstrate the immense complexity of human behavior. A range of biological, social and psychological factors are known to relate to behavior both directly and indirectly through complex interactions within interdependent systems (Engel, 1977). Within much of psychology and sociology there has been an emphasis on mental and emotional activities and processes. Sociologists talk about beliefs, values, feelings, experiences and meanings, whereas psychologists tend to talk in terms of cognition, affect and volition. Precise definitions of these concepts are less important than recognition of the wide disciplinary agreement that people's beliefs, attitudes and mental processes, however defined, influence their behavior. Clearly, other factors have been shown to relate to behavior, including biological influences, age, gender and social factors, such as poverty. Why then the emphasis on these rather than other factors? The answer is simply that research has suggested that they are not only accessible but also open to a degree of change. Indeed there is evidence that health interventions that are based on an acknowledgement of patients' views, identified through social cognition approaches in particular, are more effective than others (Norman *et al.*, 2000). This is not to say that change is easy to attain, or that it is necessarily desirable in all cases. In identifying the underlying beliefs and rationale that underpin *non-compliance*, a clinician might find him- or herself in agreement with the patient that perhaps in their circumstances and with their desired endpoints their *non-compliant* medication-taking behavior *is* the best option.

Taking a cognitive approach is highly compatible with the underlying values of the patient-centered approach. It seeks to understand people by identifying their values, hopes, fears and concerns. This approach also facilitates a respect for the autonomy of individuals and the right that they have to pursue their goals, yet it can open up a dialogue within which such goals can be examined, adjusted, redefined or simply pursued.

Although psychologists, sociologists and anthropologists have all been involved in identifying and describing beliefs relating to medication-taking behavior, it is predominantly health psychologists who have categorized such cognitive processes into both heuristic and predictive models. The remainder of this chapter will concentrate on describing a number of these models and their relevance for understanding medication-taking behavior and aiding patient-centered prescribing. However, prior to this it is worth making the point that the models should not be thought of as fully complete, definitive or static. We are not claiming that they embody a universal and long-lasting truth or formula, but rather they are *models* – simplified representations to help us to make sense of the highly complex reality that is human behavior. They are best assessed in terms of their usefulness for a given task. This may be the predictive ability that they provide, the effectiveness of interventions that are based on them, or even the extra empathy that they may help the clinician to gain with his or her patient. Clinicians may find them useful as a map to inform discussions with patients and to attempt to clarify their hopes, fears and potential goals. For instance, many will be familiar with the notion that an event such as a heart attack can be a useful cue for stopping smoking, and that cognisant professionals can make use of this opportunity.

The remainder of this chapter will examine four behavior models, all of which have been used to explore, understand, predict and research medication taking, especially the cognitive component (or the 'intentional' aspect of *non-compliance*). However, rather than seeing these models as in competition with each other, it may be more useful to consider the importance and relevance of each (and its constituent parts) in the light of a given clinical situation. No one model holds the truth. Indeed there is ongoing interest in trying to harmonize the varying models to form a summary model that can be used for more clinical purposes. Abraham and Sheeran (2000) have recently commented that the identification of a summary model that could highlight common theoretical understandings of the cognitive antecedents of motivation but could also include behavior-specific antecedents would be extremely useful.

Ley's cognitive hypothesis model

Ley's model was originally designed to help to understand *compliance* (Ley, 1982). Ley postulated that *compliance* stemmed from both an individual's recall of medical advice, and their understanding of the content of a consultation, including the doctor's explanation of the clinical problem and the rationale for the treatment. He suggested that not only would these two factors influence medication taking directly, but also they would have a further impact, albeit indirectly, through patient satisfaction with the doctor and the consultation in general.

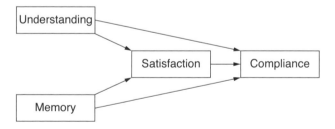

Figure 4.1   Ley's model of compliance.

Memory

It has been known for a long time that many patients cannot recall key elements of advice from the consultation. In 1977, Bain conducted a study among patients attending a family doctor in the UK. A third of the patients could not recall the name of the drug they were receiving, a quarter could not recall the length of time for which they should continue treatment, and a further quarter could not remember the dose. The more complex the prescribed regimen, the greater the likelihood that memory will fail and errors will result (Ley, 1983; Finn and Alcorn, 1986; Pullar *et al.*, 1988), despite the fact that most information can be obtained simply by reading the instructions on the bottle. Memory and complexity of the regimen may be the type of problem that many health professionals prefer, as this 'accidental' misuse assumes that the patient had intended to take their medication, so time and effort probably do not need to be spent cajoling the individual into changing their views. Furthermore, although not simple, recall is one of the more easily grasped problems to address. Dose-dispensing units, reminders and enhancing the role of family members have all been successfully employed to address such recall problems (Rehder *et al.*, 1980; Walker, 1992).

Understanding

For a patient to take medication as prescribed, they clearly need to understand what that recommendation is. Furthermore, unless they are in a totally deferential relationship with the clinician (an increasingly unlikely scenario), they will probably need some understanding of the rationale underlying the doctor's recommendation. Such an understanding may include a model of the underlying disease process, the organs that are affected and the way in which the suggested treatment can address this. However, achieving such an understanding may be problematic even if the clinician has excellent communication skills. Patients will bring their own understanding of anatomy, physiology and language to the consultation, however accurate or inaccurate this may be, and they may use medical terminology in very different ways from clinicians. Pearson and Dudley (1982) found that of 729 survey responses in which members of the public were asked to locate major body organs, 28% were correct, 14% gave vague indications of location and 58% were incorrect. In terms of physiology, a frequently cited lay example is the 'plumbing model' of the human body (Kleinman *et al.*, 1978). This may be used by many patients as a framework to aid understanding through a process of visualization. For example, Kleinman has described how the plumbing model has informed one folk belief about constipation. Understanding of constipation as 'blocked bowels' is regarded as potentially hazardous, since faeces that are retained within the bowel are visualized as diffusing into the bloodstream, thereby endangering health.

While models of lay anatomy and physiology can be a source of misunderstanding, they may also provide useful metaphors through which clinicians can communicate complex ideas, such as physiological processes. However, they can also be an obstacle, particularly if they are not elucidated. For example, Williams (1983) has reported the existence of different conceptualizations of mental health problems. Many people have a strongly 'social' model of depression, according to which social pressures and events of varying severity build up or coincide within a short time period, creating 'pressure' or 'wearing down' an individual's resistance or inner strength. However, for these individuals such a model makes it difficult to see antidepressants as a solution. Since the cause is not biological, how can a chemical help? If the antidepressant is taken, it may well be perceived as simply addressing the symptoms rather than the illness or the cause of the illness. The drug becomes a 'crutch', and is seen as a symbol of the patient's inability to cope with the pressures and problems of life.

Satisfaction

There have been various criticisms of the concept of satisfaction. Central to these is the question of whether it fully or meaningfully embodies patients' views of medical care (Williams, 1994; Avis *et al.*, 1997). Despite these concerns, there is broad agreement that it can be influenced by the consultation, and that dissatisfaction can lead to numerous forms of *non-compliance*, including medication taking. For example, Wilson and McNamara (1982) have demonstrated that perceptions of physician–patient interaction can influence satisfaction and behavioral intentions to use treatment. More recently, in a study of diet in 840 renal patients, Coyne *et al.* (1995) found that satisfaction with diet was significantly associated with dietary *compliance*.

Ley's cognitive hypothesis model is frequently cited in standard textbooks in relation to medication-taking behavior (Sarafino, 1994; Ogden, 1996). Furthermore, it is simple and easy to remember and thus potentially useful for informing discussions within a consultation. However, the simplicity of the model is also its potential weakness. It leaves the mechanisms by which understanding is derived unexplained, and does not account for what may determine satisfaction or dissatisfaction. Furthermore, although both satisfaction and understanding may relate to a person's intentions, the actual act of medication taking is not necessarily a straightforward consequence. For example, in a review of the effectiveness of educational interventions, Raynor (1992) found that although leaflets can increase both satisfaction and patient knowledge, they may have little actual effect on *compliance*. The reason for these results is unclear. However, one explanation may be that different behaviors can be induced by either dissatisfaction or satisfaction, and that these, rather than being two ends of a continuum, are in fact conceptually different phenomena (Coyle 1997, 1999). Ley's model may therefore be too simplistic to be widely applicable.

Leventhal's self-regulatory model of illness behavior

In the early 1980s, Leventhal and colleagues proposed another model to expand understanding of medication taking. This could be used to help to deconstruct the origins of people's knowledge and understanding of their illness. Leventhal argued that coping with and managing an illness is a problem-solving task (Leventhal *et al.*, 1980; Leventhal and Nerenz, 1985). Individuals perceive a change in their normal bodily or mental status and are then motivated to identify the cause and nature of this departure and act to reverse the event in order to bring themselves back to their norm. Leventhal suggested that this 'self-regulatory' process consisted of three stages, namely identification and interpretation of the problem, coping with the problem, and finally an appraisal of the effectiveness of the coping strategy adopted.

Illness representations

At the heart of Leventhal's model are illness cognitions, also referred to as health or illness beliefs, or illness representations. These are people's 'common-sense' beliefs about an illness, which may derive from past knowledge or experience, relevant consultations, or conversations with family or friends. These beliefs are usually generated in response to a particular episode of illness, and may not be the same as the sufferer's beliefs prior to the onset of illness. A range of research studies on numerous disease topics has suggested that these illness beliefs can be grouped into five categories or 'dimensions':

- **identity**: the name of the illness and its constituent nature (e.g. symptomatology)
- **perceived cause**: the physical, social, psychological or even spiritual cause of the illness

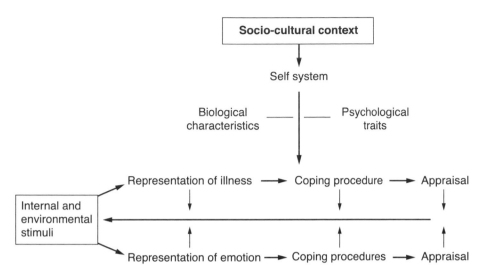

Figure 4.2 Self-regulatory model of illness. Taken from Horne and Weinman (2000).

- **consequences**: the likely impact of the illness on the individual – this may be physical, psychological or social
- **time line:** the expected duration of the illness – acute or chronic
- **curability and controllability**: the extent to which the person believes that the illness can be cured or controlled either by him- or herself or by a qualified other.

There is strong empirical evidence to support the content of these five dimensions (Lau and Hartman, 1983; Bishop and Converse, 1986; Skinner and Hampson, 2001; Skinner *et al.*, 2002) and to suggest that they are useful both heuristically and as a predictor of future illness behavior. Weinman has conducted a significant amount of research using Leventhal's concept of illness representation as the basis of the Illness Perception Questionnaire (IPQ) in order to understand a range of illness behaviors (Weinman *et al.*, 1996). A number of disease-specific versions of the IPQ have now been developed, including arthritis, diabetes and chronic fatigue syndrome.

Horne has recently demonstrated a link between Leventhal's dimensions of illness beliefs and medication taking among people with hypertension (Horne *et al.*, 2001). In addition, there is evidence that individuals who have experienced an episode of heart disease have difficulties in establishing and maintaining self-care, due to problematic illness cognitions (Karner *et al.*, 2002). A qualitative study by Wiles and Kinmonth (2001) found that patients' willingness to adopt secondary preventive strategies following a heart attack was influenced by their understanding of their condition. The data suggested that information received from health professionals encouraged patients to view a heart attack as an acute event rather than as a symptom of a chronic condition, and that this understanding provided patients with low motivation for long-term lifestyle change. The concept of illness representations has also been used to inform methods of communication within primary care settings. For example, Theunissen *et al.* (2003) conducted a three-armed experimental study to examine whether action plans relating to hypertension could be influenced by discussing patients' illness beliefs within a clinical consultation. A total of 108 patients with hypertension were involved, and the different types of conversations were found to affect some of the patients' ideas and plans.

There is widespread support for Leventhal's idea that people conceptualize illness beliefs along these five dimensions. Researchers in other disciplinary areas have worked along similar lines and generated similar, although not identical conceptualizations. For example, the anthropologist Arthur Kleinman has argued that it is possible to identify 'explanatory models' (EMs) which encompass notions about an episode of sickness and its treatment (Kleinman, 1980; Young, 1981). These models typically encompass:

- the aetiology or cause of the condition
- the timing and mode of onset of symptoms
- the pathophysiological processes involved
- the natural history and severity of the illness
- the appropriate treatments for the condition.

Such models also exist among both health professionals and the general public, and have been identified and described for a range of clinical conditions and 'folk illnesses' (Rubel, 1977). Kleinman went on to suggest the following standard questions that may be used to elicit these underlying explanatory models.

1 What do you call the problem?
2 What do you think has caused the problem?
3 Why do you think it started when it did?
4 What do you think the sickness does? How does it work?
5 How severe is the sickness? Will it have a short or long course?
6 What kind of treatment do you think you should receive? What are the most important results you hope to receive from this treatment?
7 What are the chief problems the sickness has caused?
8 What do you fear most about the sickness?

Health and illness beliefs may not only be important as correlates of behavior, but may also actually influence the disease process itself. For example, Hahn and Kleinman (1983) have highlighted the role that beliefs can play in creating a negative placebo effect, namely a 'nocebo' effect. Many people may consider the idea of nocebo as more relevant to developing or non-western societies than to rich or developed nations. However, nocebo may simply take different forms – the 'evil eye' in one country or culture and the equating of cancer with death in another. It has the potential to be relevant whenever a strong lay explanatory model exists. Although it has not yet been researched in detail, there remains the possibility that the nocebo effect has an impact on medication use whenever, rightly or wrongly, there are strong beliefs about side-effects. Indeed Leventhal's or Kleinman's dimensions could be used to explore a patient's beliefs about perceived side-effects of medication as well as symptoms of an illness.

Stage 1: Interpretation

Leventhal suggested that the interpretation of a deviation from a normal state depends on both a recognition of a change and the application of a set of beliefs to those symptoms. The recognition may be by the individual him- or herself (symptom perception) and/or through social messages (from friends, family or indeed the clinician). There is then a parallel reaction through the creation of both a cognitive representation of the problem and an affective response. The initial interpretation is then likely to result in an emotional response, which in turn can affect the symptom interpretation. For example, a pregnant woman may have experienced postnatal depression after the birth of her first child. Soon after the arrival of her second child, she begins to notice the symptoms of depression again (symptom perception), and her husband also notices them and expresses some concern (social messages). The recognition and interpretation of the symptoms as the return of postnatal depression will then produce a further emotional reaction (fear, anxiety, etc.).

Stage 2: Coping

The identification, interpretation and emotional response provide the motivation for either action or inaction, including either taking medication or refusing it. Within the Leventhal model, coping strategies are required to address both the cognitive process and the affective response. The nature and range of possible strategies is not covered in detail in the Leventhal model, although some authors have made a distinction between avoidance and approach coping as broad strategies or typologies (Ogden, 1996). These conceptualizations are too broad to be of much use. However, the literature on coping itself may prove extremely useful within the context of attempts to move towards patient-centered prescribing.

Any clinician who provides treatment will become part of the patient's coping strategy. The concordance model and the idea of a therapeutic alliance suggest that a partnership is developed through negotiation concerning a common interpretation of existing problems and a common set of goals (Royal Pharmaceutical Society of Great Britain, 1997). For the prescriber, the question is how the goals can be achieved and whether a strategy can be agreed upon and implemented.

While Leventhal has highlighted the problem-solving focus of illness behavior, other work by Moos and Swindle has highlighted three coping processes that may be employed in relation to such problems. These are cognitive appraisal, adaptive tasks and coping skills (Moos and Swindle, 1984). Cognitive appraisal is sufficiently similar to stage 1 of Leventhal's model to require little coverage here. Specifically, Moos and Swindle argued that at the onset of an illness, or an acute episode within the context of a chronic illness, there is likely to be an appraisal of the severity of the situation. This severity may not simply relate to issues of symptoms, morbidity or likely mortality, but to the social and psychological consequences of both illness and treatments as well. Ogden has suggested that Leventhal's illness representations can be integrated into this cognitive appraisal stage, as such illness beliefs are integral to how an illness will be appraised (Ogden, 1996). Having a framework through which the patient's appraisal may be accessed may be particularly important when the experience of an illness may be far removed from the personal experience of the clinician. For example, Rubenstein has provided a graphic account of the onset of multiple sclerosis and highlighted a range of experiences that could be difficult to imagine or empathize with from an outsider's perspective. These include a sense of powerlessness, a new dependence on doctors and technology, and a sense of 'not being quite human anymore' (Rubenstein, 1985).

Adaptive tasks

Once there has been an appraisal of the illness, Moos and Swindle suggest that seven tasks falling into two categories might be engaged in. Again, this taxonomy may provide a useful framework for considering the likely relationship between the patient's goals and decisions about medication taking.

General tasks

1 Preparing for the future.
2 Preserving self-image, competence and mastery.
3 Maintaining relationships with family and friends.
4 Preserving an emotional balance.

Illness-related tasks

1 Dealing with pain and other symptoms.
2 Dealing with treatment environment or procedures (including medication).
3 Developing and maintaining relationships with health professionals.

Within a patient-centered paradigm, medication should ideally be considered and discussed in relation to each of the above. Any drug regimen may impact on a variety of tasks and include trade-off that it may help to discuss. For example, with regard to general tasks, a young boy with exercise-induced asthma may prepare for the future by considering inhaler use and the degree to which it can facilitate exercise participation and thus maintain his relationships with family and friends. However, he may also find that the explicit dependence on and overt use of the inhaler can damage his self-image and undermine his emotional balance.

   Although some authors have made attempts to integrate the work mentioned above, the size and nature of the model would be too large and comprehensive to bring to mind in the clinical setting. However, the work of Leventhal, Kleinman, Moos and Schaefer among others points to four main issues of which practitioners should be aware when attempting to comprehend their patients' perspectives.

1 People experience, interpret and attribute bodily symptoms, and they use frameworks to do so.
2 These interpretations will profoundly influence their responses (and therefore only a foolish clinician ignores them).
3 They actively appraise and problem solve.
4 This includes seeking emotional resolution as well as cognitive solutions.

Leventhal's model and patient-centered prescribing

Leventhal's model and its self-regulatory, problem-focussed foundation may prove useful for practitioners who wish to gain an insight into the move towards more patient-centered prescribing. The strength of Leventhal's model is its linking of beliefs to an emotional reaction and subsequently through to a behavior. If a practitioner can gain an insight into the specific details of a patient's beliefs about their illness (what they think it is, what caused it, how long it will last, its consequences and whether it is curable) *and* the emotional reaction in terms of its nature (anger, fear, despair, etc.), their reactions suddenly become more understandable. This can help at a number of levels.

Facilitating empathy

Since the doctor and patient roles are now dramatically changing from historical deferential patterns, a new foundation is required for the relationship. The patient-centered model strongly implies that each party brings something unique to the consultation. The patient brings their illness, interpretation, problems and values, while the doctor brings both knowledge and skill with regard to the interpretation of cause and potential cures. If a degree of concordance between the respective parties is to be achieved, there must be an understanding of each other's perspectives and, hopefully through consultation, eventual agreement on a common interpretation, goal and course of action. For the doctor, at least initially, this means trying to get 'into the patient's shoes', to see the problem through their eyes (Gerteis *et al.*, 1993). If this can be achieved then the empathy that is generated can form a basis for a productive doctor–patient relationship. Indeed this is the foundation of motivational interviewing. Rollnick *et al.* (1999) have suggested that empathy is a prerequisite for any meaningful communication that aims to clarify dilemmas from a patient's perspective ('discrepancy' in the motivational interviewing nomenclature). Leventhal's concept of illness representations and its constituent dimensions are useful frameworks for helping the prescriber to uncover and comprehend the thinking underlying a patient's behavior (Theunissen *et al.*, 2003).

Symptom/side-effect interpretation

Symptom perception is problematic. There is evidence that some patients overestimate their ability to detect symptoms. Such false detection or interpretation may lead to inappropriate decisions about medication use. Skelton and Pennebaker (1982) have pointed to the role of cognitions, mood and environment in influencing the experience and interpretation of internal body states. For example, there is now a body of evidence showing that people with hypertension frequently overestimate their ability to detect raised blood pressure. These individuals tend to cite a set of internal body cues such as dizziness, headaches or nervousness that correlate more closely with symptoms and mood than with blood pressure itself (Pennebaker and Watson, 1988; Watson and Pennebaker, 1989).

So what is the relevance for patient-centered prescribing of symptom interpretation being problematic? Being patient-centered should not mean simply adopting the immediate perspective of the patient and acting as a mechanic, merely called in to 'fix the problem' as recognized and interpreted by the patient. The interpretation is open to negotiation, depending on the individual's illness beliefs, symptom perception and emotional response to their situation. This may mean satisfactorily explaining an experience (such as normal but often alarming nodular breast development in adolescent boys) or, in some cases, it may provide an interpretation that produces fear or anxiety for the patient. For example, Pennebaker's conclusion regarding people's inability to estimate their own blood pressure was that 'if these erroneous beliefs can be eliminated, subjects may be able to estimate BP fluctuations more accurately' (Pennebaker and Watson, 1988). However, such a process may well cause anxiety, as an element of previously perceived control is lost.

Symptom interpretation will clearly involve both recognition of a phenomenon and an interpretation based on an assessment of normal variation in body experience, progression with age, a disease, or the side-effect of a drug, among other factors. Again, the prescriber can have a role at this stage when a likely cause is being established. In a recently conducted study of clozapine use by people with treatment-resistant schizophrenia, a number of individuals who had shown significant clinical improvements were found to attribute what may have been 'normal' experiences to their medication. These ongoing problems tended to centre on drowsiness/lethargy, poor motivation and lack of clear thinking or a 'fuzzy head.' Some individuals tended to attribute these problems to their medication, although there was every possibility that they were experiencing everyday variations in mood and function. The most commonly reported experience was 'laziness', which commonly appeared to be of a fairly normal nature.

Case example: Jack

> Interviewer: "Okay. Well, we've sort of asked you a wee bit about being in hospital. You started on clozapine and you're sort of quite a bit down the line now. Is it causing you any more difficulties or problems?"
> Jack: "No, it makes me quite lazy like. I just sit and stare at the TV when I should be practicing my scales and practicing chords and ... just practicing so I'm getting my cool thing back together again."
> Interviewer: "Is there anything that you do that helps you to deal with that tiredness?"
> Jack: "Go out for walks like. I get a good half hour/hour walk every day, or thereabouts."

The health belief model

Although the health belief model (Becker *et al.*, 1977) is predominantly a model of health behaviors (e.g. diet, exercise, etc.), it has been used with some success to help to understand and predict some forms of illness behavior, such as medication taking (Bond *et al.*, 1992; Budd *et al.*, 1996; Brown and Segal, 1997; Hughes *et al.*, 1997). The content has some overlap with Leventhal's model, but includes a number of different concepts.

The health belief model incorporates four main precursors to behavior, namely threat perception, behavioral evaluation, cues to action and health motivation. Threat perception can be broken down into the perceived severity of an illness or event and the perceived susceptibility to (likelihood of) the illness or event. For example, in the context of medication, consider a person with a history of epilepsy. The perceived health threat would be at its highest (and the person would be *more* likely to take medication) when they perceive a seizure to be serious in biological, social and/or psychological terms *and* they perceive the likelihood of a seizure as being significant. If either of these are absent, there would be minimal gain from taking preventive action. Perceptions of

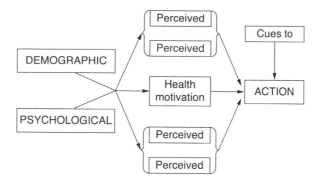

Figure 4.3 The health belief model.

severity may stem from underlying health/illness beliefs, past experience or the likely social context in which an event may take place (e.g. in public or while riding a bike). Perceptions of susceptibility are again likely to stem from past experience and underlying health beliefs, both of these components having clear parallels in Leventhal's 'representation of illness.'

Behavioral evaluation consists of an assessment of the benefits of the action and the corresponding costs of or barriers to that action. Again, in the context of medication taking, behavioral evaluation would be at its lowest when an individual believes that the benefit is low (i.e. the drug is relatively ineffective) and the costs are high (e.g. significant side-effects, financial cost, lack of availability of the drug). Again there are parallels in the sense of a judgement call being required. Of course, one common difference with preventive actions is that there is no event if they have succeeded, so they cannot be judged against more concrete factors such as symptoms. For instance, patients with atrial fibrillation (a heart arrhythmia) are currently asked to consider taking warfarin as an anticoagulant to prevent a stroke. However, whatever the outcome, they can never know whether their decision was the right one for them. Such risk appraisal is more common in preventive care than in more obviously therapeutic interventions.

Cues to action can refer to a range of discrete events that may prompt the individual to change his or her behavior. These may include the onset of a particular symptom, an adverse event happening to a friend, the impact of advice or health education campaigns, or indeed a consultation with a doctor. A final influence on behavior that was not in the original versions of the health belief model is health motivation. This reflected people's general readiness to be concerned about health. However, health motivation has had far less attention paid to it than other components of the model, and its influence on medication taking has been little explored.

Although the health belief model highlights some important conceptual areas that may be worthy of discussion and consideration in the clinical encounter, it has a number of critics. One problem has been the lack of a robust research evidence base to support the model as a whole. In 1992, Harrison *et al.* conducted a meta-analysis of the relationships between four dimensions of the health belief model (*susceptibility, severity, benefits* and *costs*) and health behavior in 16 studies that measured all four of the dimensions and their relationship to behavioral variables. The results showed limited support for the model as whole. The weak effect of sizes and lack of homogeneity indicated that it was premature to draw conclusions about the predictive validity of the health belief model as employed in these studies. However, the authors highlighted the fact that the finding of only 16 studies which met the minimum criteria for valid representation of the dimensions of the health belief model indicates that future studies should focus more on such issues.

The theory of planned behavior

The final model that will be considered here is the theory of planned behavior (Ajzen, 1985, 1991). This theory has been used to predict an impressively wide array of behaviors – from kidney donation, through driving behaviors to visiting public houses. Among these there are studies of medication taking. One clear clinical example has concerned mothers' intentions to use oral rehydration therapy (Hounsa *et al.*, 1993).

There are three elements of the theory of planned behavior that are relevant to medication taking and are not specifically included in the health belief model or self-regulatory model. These are subjective norm, self-efficacy/perceived behavioral control, and intentions. The following example may help to illustrate the nature and importance of these concepts.

Case example: John

Consider John, a 50-year-old man with hypertension who is asymptomatic, does not feel ill, does not regard raised blood pressure as a major problem and does not feel particularly susceptible to any subsequent adverse events. While he does not really perceive any benefits from taking antihypertensives, he equally does not see any harm in taking them. He has a history of taking his drugs religiously, but why? His wife, whose father had hypertension and died in his late forties, is concerned about her husband's health. She has expressed this concern to him along with her view that he should take his drugs, which she sets out for him each morning. The health belief model does not give explicit place to the views of others such as this. The theory of planned behavior refers to these views as 'subjective norms.' The theory proposes that a person's perceptions of what others think he or she should do *and* the degree to which that person values the views of those others will together influence subsequent health or illness behavior.

Another element of the theory of planned behavior that overlaps to some degree with the barrier concept within the health belief model is perceived behavioral control – or an individual's beliefs that they are able to engage in the behavior. For example, a person with insulin-dependent diabetes may recognize the importance of good blood sugar control, but find it extremely difficult to cope with needles or finger pricks. Such beliefs about the ability to perform actions have been found to stem from both internal and external factors. Internal factors relate to issues of knowledge, memory and skill, while external factors refer to the availability of the resources, such as treatment or the ability to pay for it.

While previous models of health and illness behavior attempted to relate cognitions to subsequent behavior, many researchers questioned how attitudes and beliefs come to be transformed into behavior. Fishbein and Ajzen (1975) argued that this process included the creation of intentions, and that cognitions are better predictors of intention than of

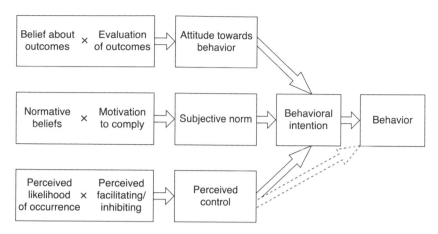

Figure 4.4 Theory of planned behavior.

behavior directly. However, it should be noted that since intentions are a conscious creation, they relate only to what might be termed 'volitional behaviors', and would exclude highly routine acts. Ajzen (1991) found that, when applied across a range of behaviors, there is a relatively strong and consistent correlation (0.7) between underlying cognitions in the theory of planned behavior and intentions. However, the relationship between intentions and actual behavior is more problematic, with correlations ranging from 0.1 to 0.94 (Sheppard *et al.*, 1988). One of the underlying theoretical bases for the theory of planned behavior is the principle of 'compatibility' (Fishbein and Ajzen, 1975). This is worth considering in more detail. The principle suggests that attitudes and behaviors have four elements, namely action, context, target and time. The greatest correspondence between attitudes and behavior will exist when they are matched in terms of specificity. In other words, attitudes will lead to behaviors which consist of an action that is performed on a target in a particular context and at a specific time. In terms of medication taking, a patient may take one medication (action and target) at home (context) each morning (time), but they might apply a different attitude (intention) to another medication (Conner and Sparks, 1996).

Research on the volitional process – that is, how intentions come to be transformed into behavior – has received less attention than other aspects of the theory of planned behavior. However, Gollwitzer (1993a,b) has made a useful distinction between goal intentions and implementation intentions. He suggests that individuals may have a broad intention to engage in a particular behavior, but that this lacks details and specificity. Implementation intentions refer to the details of how the goal intention is to be translated. They include how, where and in what circumstances the behavior will be engaged in. For example, a person with chronic asthma may intend to use their inhaler in order to prevent attacks (goal intention). On its own this intention is so broad (few details have been decided upon with regard to how and when the behavior will be engaged in) that it may well not take place. However, if the person or doctor suggests that the inhaler is used every morning just before brushing their teeth (to rinse residue from the throat), the detail and association with tooth brushing (acting as a cue to action) may increase the likelihood of the behavior occurring. Clearly there is a role here for prescribers in enabling patients in the volitional process of effectively implementing their own intentions.

There are two lessons here for practitioners of patient-centered prescribing. First, there is reassurance that by exploring the underlying issues embodied in the theory of planned behavior, a good indication and possibly understanding of intention may be derived. Secondly, patients may wish and indeed intend to follow a prescribed regimen, but the problem may be related to actual control over the behavior itself. In other words, where intentions do not appear to result in behavior this may be because they are frustrated by lack of skills, opportunities or resources, or even by a poor memory. This, of course, brings the argument full circle. Such 'accidental' misuse is just as important as its more intriguing partner, and patient-centered prescribers still need to be able to focus on enabling the patient to implement their intentions to take medication.

Multidimensional health locus of control

While the theory of planned behavior contains the notion of perceived behavioral control, it was pre-dated by a wider concept known as *health locus of control (HLC)*. Rotter provided the theoretical foundation for the concept through social learning theory in the 1950s (Rotter, 1954). The central tenet of social learning theory is that the likelihood of a behavior occurring in a given situation is a function of the individual's expectation that the behavior will lead to a particular outcome *and* the extent to which that outcome is valued. Locus of control was therefore seen in one-dimensional terms, as the degree to which an individual believed that control over a particular event lay with him- or herself (internal) or elsewhere (external). This original scale had some limited success in predicting health behaviors (Strickland, 1978). However, the amount of variance was low, and many researchers thought that the construct was too basic. This concept was therefore later refined into the *multidimensional health locus of control (MHLC)*, in which external control was subdivided into either 'powerful others' or 'chance/fate.' In terms of medication taking, this distinction might be illustrated by considering two patients. One patient is willing to take their medication, and in fact demands a significant amount of information about the drug, its side-effects and optimum doses. This patient believes that the future of their illness lies with them and their behavior (internal locus of control). Another patient may refuse medication and simply say 'If I'm going to get worse then I'm going to get worse – there's nothing I can do about it' (external – chance/fate).

The MHLC has been used in a large number of studies to predict health behaviors. However, while there appear to be good theoretical and common-sense reasons why individuals who do not think their illness is within their control should be less adherent, there is a paucity of empirical evidence. Even the research relating to health behaviors such as exercise and smoking has proved weak or inconsistent (Calnan, 1989). Norman and Bennett (1998) have reviewed the history and use of the HLC and subsequent MHLC. In particular, they considered its relationship to exercise, alcohol, smoking, AIDS-related behavior, breast self-examination, smoking cessation and weight loss. For each topic they comment that there are conflicting findings and/or only weak associations.

One criticism made of the MHLC is that it will only predict health behavior if an individual values health. In other words, perception of internal control will only lead to a behavior if the endpoint of that behavior is valued. In addition, the scale that is widely used to measure MHLC may be too general. Ajzen and Fishbein (1977) have argued that *specific* attitudes/beliefs are more likely to lead to *specific* behavior, and many studies looking at MHLC have used a general attitude to predict a specific behavior. There has therefore been a move to try to develop behavior-specific scales of HLC (Norman and Bennett, 1998). This has met with more success. For example, Georgiou and Bradley (1992) developed a smoking-specific locus of control scale to examine smokers' beliefs about quitting. This scale was found to have greater predictive validity than the general scale, and people with an internal locus of control were found to quit for longer periods of time.

Although there is a dearth of studies relating locus of control to medication taking, one study has provided interesting and relevant findings. A study of 551 women diagnosed with breast cancer in Portland, Oregon found that individuals with a high internal locus of control were more likely to take their care into their own hands and use complementary and alternative medicines (Henderson and Donatelle, 2003). Consequently, a reluctance or refusal to take medication may stem from either internal or external loci of control.

There is a need for further research to examine the relationship between MHLC and medication use. However, the notion that individuals may perceive control over their medication and illness differently, and that these differences may influence decisions about medication taking, appears sensible and straightforward and should probably be considered within the consultation.

Final comments

The purpose of this chapter has been to use current theoretical and empirical research to highlight the varied attitudes and beliefs that may influence an individual's medication-taking behaviors and indicate the complexity of their origins. It has not sought to provide a detailed academic account of the contemporary state of play in behavioral research. The components of attitudes and values that are described above are likely to be a significant component of the discussion within any patient-centered prescribing process. A prior knowledge of what they may be is likely to help in unearthing them and in raising their importance for patients. Although the range of issues contained within the various models (perceived severity, susceptibility, self-efficacy, intentions, etc.) can be somewhat bewildering, these models provide a heuristic device that represents the current state of the art, imperfect as this may be. They should not be regarded as definitive, and research is continuing in all areas of their application. Issues others than those currently identified in the literature will arise in many consultations, and it is important that the clinician is not blinded to their existence by an over-reliance on fitting the patient's views into some pre-existing conceptual framework.

The models have been presented to help to identify each unique pattern of hopes, fears, concerns, values and beliefs in relation to the prescribing process. However, there are also calls for the integration of the various models (Shaw, 1999; Abraham and Sheeran, 2000), and by definition a patient-centered approach should be 'realistic' in nature. At present there is no common and uniform model that has been agreed upon within the behavioral science community. The problem for practitioners, therefore, is which model to use to inform their prescribing practices, when each clearly has its own strengths and weaknesses. The following chapter proposes a model that may be more conducive to this while retaining the key components and processes identified so far.

Conclusion

In Chapter 4 we have considered the need to assimilate the patient's beliefs and external influences with models that might help us to understand how behaviors are influenced as a result. It is this understanding that suggests how we might best seek to influence these behaviors, assuming that this is a legitimate aim. This is comparable with a molecular chemist who seeks to design a drug based upon a thorough understanding of the various pathways on which it needs to act, or indeed avoid acting, in order to have the desired effect. Rather than testing thousands of potential compounds, it is increasingly possible to build molecules of the correct shape. Sometimes even one isomer (mirror image) is known to be active, and drug effects can be enhanced by selecting out only this active half of the preparation. In the same way, it should be possible to design and fine-tune interventions to alter the way in which an illness is conceived, or the way in which a risk is perceived, or the way in which a medicine's effect is interpreted. Although we understand the behavioral systems less well than many of the physiological ones, we have the opportunity to tailor the intervention to each individual. When Balint coined the phrase 'Doctor as drug', he had this notion in mind. With enough knowledge and skill, we should be able to identify and push enough of the right buttons to have an impact. The next chapter aims to help you to identify the buttons through conversations with your patients.

The patient-centered prescribing process

Chapter 5

Decision making and the patient's voice: the therapeutic decision model

Brian Williams and Jon Dowell

Introduction

This chapter seeks to bring together the various concepts and models that have been presented in Chapters 3 and 4 in a simplified format that makes sense to clinicians and can be related directly to individual patients. To do this, we offer a unified model, the *therapeutic decision model*. This forms the basis for understanding how patients engage with clinicians and others when having to make decisions about treatment, and therefore the consultation techniques described in the next two chapters.

The previous chapters highlighted a range of practical and conceptual issues that have been found to influence attitudes to and the action of medication taking. Earlier chapters provided the patient's perspective, but in a second-hand fashion and through different conceptual lenses. However, there are also calls for the integration of the various models (Shaw, 1999; Abraham and Sheeran, 2000), and by definition a patient-centered approach should be 'realistic' in nature. Therefore this chapter seeks to provide a unifying model that is more easily grasped by clinicians. We illustrate the model through the use of patients' stories and quotes. These are given to help readers to link these abstract concepts with clinical practice. We have chosen to present these accounts alongside the therapeutic decision model (TDM) because clinicians are familiar with process models (how someone may consider a drug, try it out, and modify their views and then their behavior), and a more comprehensive single model appears to be lacking. This particular model was designed to incorporate the key elements, all those pertinent to medication use (and presented in Chapter 4) and the findings of qualitative research designed to analyse this issue afresh (Dowell and Hudson, 1997). Although it has been assimilated from established conceptual models, this has been done in a novel way that has yet to be critically tested. To provide some supportive evidence, we describe a number of real cases to illustrate how the TDM accords with clinical experience.

We should pause here, however, to consider the value and purpose of using patients' stories and accounts to form the link to practice. While it may be impossible to truly stand in someone else's shoes, researchers and authors generally have used stories or narratives as a way of allowing insights into the nature of these experiences. Of course the level of success varies according to the skills of the author or narrator. However, the subject matter also comes into play. For example, beliefs may be understood relatively easily, whereas gaining insight into more abstract and existential issues such as 'suffering' is always likely to be difficult (Frank, 2001).

The renowned work of Arthur Kleinman (Kleinman, 1988) and Arthur Frank (Frank, 1995) has demonstrated the power of people's stories, and recently the medical press has begun to popularize the use of the narrative for approaching a patient's problems holistically and uncovering diagnostic and therapeutic options (Greenhalgh and Hurwitz, 1988). At the same time, the public has been receptive to accounts written or co-written by sporting or media celebrities. Lance Armstrong's battle with cancer (Armstrong, 2001) and William Styron's experience of depression (Styron, 2001) both give insights into the experience of illness and the perspective of the sufferer that would be missing from the more objective, standardized and conceptual accounts embodied in the models outlined in the previous chapter.

So what is the relationship between the behavioral models outlined in Chapter 4, the popular sector described in Chapter 2, and the stories that people tell about their lives and their illnesses? A relationship must surely exist, as both are rooted in the reported experiences of patients. Narrative arguably provides the added dimension that is missing from many of the models. The movement over time, and the way in which this is interpreted, remembered and reported by the individual patient, can be highly informative. The concepts in the models can be seen as ingredients that make up the story – they are the characters and the plot. The illness beliefs set the scene against which the plot (coping mechanism and appraisal process) develops (Leventhal *et al.*, 1980; Leventhal and Nerenz, 1985). The impact and consequent reinterpretation of the situation hint at future choices and provide the final act.

The therapeutic decision model

As it is derived inductively from patients' explanations in conjunction with study of existing models, the TDM reflects a range of patient narratives as well as theoretical perspectives. It therefore provides a structure for identifying the range of possible scenarios and stories that patients may see or report themselves as experiencing. Obviously patients' journeys from a perceived healthy state to being a user of any medication, or indeed rejecting treatment, may not be simple, swift or entirely linear. Sometimes new information or perhaps experience (including the results of trying out a suggested medicine) will inform the way in which the problem is seen, and this will lead to altered behavior. Such feedback loops are an essential component for all but the most trusting individuals. Hence the TDM should be seen as a simplified schematic that attempts to make sense of a dynamic and multifactorial process. Although they generally progress from left to right, individuals may recirculate many times by such internal loops before establishing a stable pattern of medication use. This is represented in Figure 5.1 by both core *consultation and testing processes* and an overarching link from *actual medication use* back to the *representation of illness and treatment*, which may of course be affected by the outcome of treatment.

So how might this model help clinicians? The TDM seeks to embody the ongoing processes of decision making, from first acknowledging that there is a health problem through to longer-term management and the range of possible categories of medication

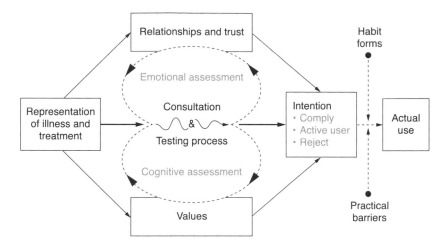

Figure 5.1 The therapeutic decision model.

users. It seeks to illustrate the process engaged in by patients as it applies to each medication, depicting how use becomes established. Even one individual may demonstrate different paths or outcomes for the different preparations they receive. Moving from the perception of the 'problem', it suggests that patients will develop an intention to act based upon their own beliefs, which may or may not be enhanced through a consultation with a doctor or other professional.

Most individuals will respond to a recommendation or prescription by trying, and in some way assessing, the treatment. Their final decision as to whether to continue using the medication or to modify or cease its use will be based upon a combination of cognitive interpretation (including the perceived likely value of the outcome) and an emotive response in terms of their desire to control their own healthcare choices and actions. Note that both of these factors may be influenced during the consultation. Patients who wish to be in control might be drawn to reject a treatment that they feel instructed to use, but might accept the same treatment if they feel that they have chosen it themselves. This is comparable to Leventhal's emotional appraisal loop and the *multiple health locus of control* theory. Even when they have decided *how* they intend to use a treatment, there is still opportunity for practical problems to intervene and reduce this further.

There are three basic routes that patients may take from left to right in this model. The two peripheral routes are very straightforward, whereas the central one is more complex. A patient with a condition that they consider to be severe but curable (e.g. pneumonia) attending a physician whom they know and trust might quickly make the decision that they can effect a cure by taking antibiotics in a compliant fashion. They might go to considerable lengths to comply – for instance, by altering diet or mealtimes as instructed, but without substantively understanding why they need to do so. In contrast, a patient with a longstanding condition (e.g. osteoarthritis) who is attending a new doctor who suggests painkillers might decide not to even try them. Their values and family norms might promote complementary and alternative medical approaches, or even soldiering on in silence without treatment. Consequently, they would reject the painkillers offered with equally little thought. However, the most complex and by far the most common scenario lies somewhere in between these two extremes. Patients often have poorly defined or tentative beliefs about their illness and treatments (Williams and Healy, 2001), and consult healthcare professionals and other sources of information as a way of clarifying these. Depending on how they view the integrity of the information source (and fortunately clinicians remain trusted more than many other members of society), they will commonly agree to at least try one or more treatment options. This testing process may provide positive reinforcement if there is an apparent benefit and relatively few drawbacks. Note that these include emotional reactions to accepting treatment, as well as symptoms and side-effects. And even these more transparent cognitive interpretations may be far from straightforward if they are based upon misconceptions about either the condition or the treatment. The patient's experiences may lead them to conclude, rightly or wrongly, that they know better than the clinician how they should use this treatment. If their understanding is incorrect, their relationship with the clinician is poor or their emotional response is negative, then it is less likely that this process will result in sustained or effective use. A typical example is the asthmatic who interprets the impact of steroid inhalers, which they may not like the sound of, on a short-term basis, and concludes that these do not work for them.

Patients' accounts

The following accounts used to illustrate the model are principally derived from four interview studies. These studies explored treatment strategies among people with treatment-resistant schizophrenia, attitudes to long-term antidepressant prescribing, the interpretation of first-onset depression, and medication use by adult primary care patients. In total they collate accounts from over 100 carefully selected respondents who were willing to provide detailed accounts of their beliefs and actions (Dowell and Hudson, 1997; Williams and Healy, 2001).

Route 1: the dominance of trust

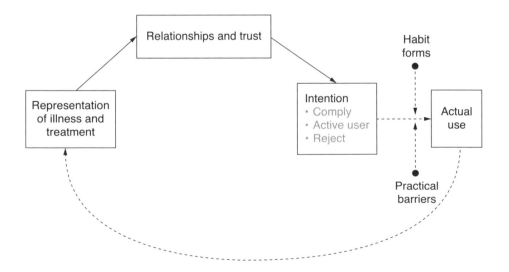

Figure 5.2   Route 1: the dominance of trust.

Case example: Rose

Rose was a 29-year-old woman with two young children who had gradually become depressed over a 6-month period. She had seen a family practitioner on a handful of occasions, but had now been referred to a psychiatrist and was awaiting a first appointment.

Illness and treatment representations: Rose began to notice that something was wrong when she realized that she was feeling and acting differently from her normal self, and when friends and family pointed out changes in her behavior.

> I was irritable, which I have never been, and a work colleague said 'You've lost the sparkle in your eyes' and other little things. I didn't want to do anything, wouldn't go out, and I was making excuses all the time. I used to say let's go here or there, and I was always first to party.

In attempting to understand these changes, Rose had considered a number of possible causes.

> I think it was my lifestyle. It's not normal and it was a lot of hard work ... my husband is away a lot ... and so it was a lot, you know. Yeah, it was probably stress. This wonderful thing we call stress.

However, an alternative explanation for her depression was the death of her parents.

> My husband said 'Oh, what do you think is the matter?' I said 'It's because of my mum and dad' [their deaths]. So, really, I think it's caught up with me now. I mean I went to see a hypnotherapist last year about my weight and ended up talking about my dad for some reason and had a good cry then. So I did feel a lot better actually after I had been to him for that. I should have just gone for my mum as well and it would have been all right. I think that's a lot of it.

Values: Since Rose's illness beliefs led her to think that the cause of her problems was a past traumatic event that had '*not been dealt with*', a biomedical solution did not seem appropriate. As a result, she attached little value to antidepressants. Instead she felt that her problems were now '*buried*' inside her mind and that they needed to be '*got out*' in some way. This led Rose to contemplate seeing a hypnotherapist in the hope that these past, hidden or buried problems could be unearthed and addressed.

Relationships and trust: Rose had a set of illness beliefs that were coherent and which made sense to her, although they also implied that a pharmaceutical solution would be inappropriate. However, these views were expressed prior to her first meeting with a psychiatrist. At that consultation the doctor recommended antidepressants and dispensed a prescription that Rose duly cashed, and she reported that she was taking the medication regularly. In a follow-up interview it was apparent that Rose's illness beliefs had not changed, although they *were* held with slightly less certainty. The value she was attaching to the medication had also changed very little. She was unsure of the rationale for the prescription or how the medication could influence what she saw as something non-biological. Nevertheless she saw the psychiatrist as the expert and trusted his experience and expertise. Rose's priority was to be rid of the depression, and this was most likely to occur by doing what the doctor had recommended, even if it did not make complete sense to her.

Intentions and actual medication use: Rose continued to take the anti-depressants over subsequent months. It took a few weeks for the medication to have an effect. However, after her depression seemed to lessen, Rose began to contemplate whether her initial view of her illness had been correct or whether it was somehow compatible with a biological solution. She sometimes wondered whether the antidepressants were simply 'masking' the depression and not actually addressing the cause. However, after 7 months she gradually reduced her dose and eventually ceased taking the medication altogether. The symptoms of her depression did not return. As a result, Rose's view of depression altered, and although it was not overly coherent, thorough or definitive, it retained the possibility of a biological origin and therefore the relevance of a pharmaceutical solution.

Case example: Gillian

Gillian was a 54-year-old married mother of two living in a small rural village. Initially she said that she was confused as to what was wrong with her. She reported having experienced a number of recent traumatic life events.

Representations of illness: Over a period of 18 months, Gillian's son had developed cancer and she herself had been involved in a fatal motor vehicle accident, and then one evening she received news that a close relative had died.

> I went to the church and some of the girls arrived and asked what was wrong. I just said 'Don't ask, because if I tell you I'll just break down again and I'll never be able to come here again.' I think things like that are bad for you – it would have been better if I had cried. I haven't been able to cry at all since then.

Gillian reported her problem as one of emotional numbness, and the symptoms that she experienced did not match her own illness beliefs about depression. As a result, she had not even considered the idea of medication.

Relationships and trust: However, although Gillian's understanding of her problem did not motivate her to take medication, she did have a very good relationship with her doctor, and sought advice from him.

> The doctor said to me 'You're suffering from depression.' Well, depression to me is when you're moping and sitting in a chair and not wanting to go out, and crying. But I'm not the doctor and he knows that there are other kinds of depression. He said that I'm weeping on the inside ... numbness, and he explained to me 'You're grieving on the inside' – which makes sense. I am quite willing to listen to that explanation.

As a result, her beliefs were changed.

Intentions and actual medication use: Gillian's views of what depression might be and might involve changed, and this led to the motivation to try antidepressants. She left the consultation with a prescription that she tried and found helpful. This assessment or informal testing process is, of course, also an important component of her account. The fact that the doctor's explanation was born out by the success of the therapy is likely to have confirmed what Gillian initially took on trust.

Route 2: the dominance of values

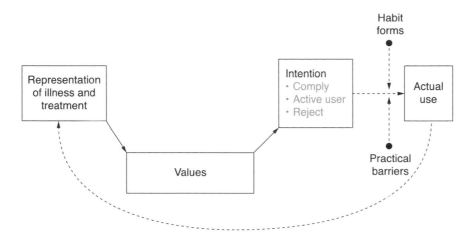

Figure 5.3   Route 2: the dominance of values.

Case example: Jane

Jane was a 25-year-old woman with a longstanding diagnosis of asthma. She lived with her fiancé and ran a riding stable.

Illness representations: Jane had suffered from asthma since the age of two and had been hospitalized many times, the most recent hospitalization being 4 years ago. She understood the cause of her condition adequately.

> Well, basically the first stage of asthma, so I've been told. I've to get an overproduction of glut and phlegm which gets into your lungs and blocks up all your tubes and then they start to narrow and you become wheezy. My lungs are just now swelling up and I'm becoming wheezy.

She found her asthma extremely unpleasant, was aware that it could be life-threatening, and acknowledged that it had limited her job prospects and social life. She perceived it as such a significant problem that she would pay '*whatever I could afford*' or risk death during surgery if a lung transplant could cure it. She also indicated that her partner would be willing to forfeit having children or to '*offer a pound of flesh*' in order to free her from asthma.

Values: Jane's understanding and her treatment approach were based on a set of values stemming from her father's and her sister's experience of asthma. This provided a motivation to '*fight it*', but not by using the recommended therapy. She chose her approach despite the fact that she had friends with asthma who had a quite different set of beliefs and management style.

> Basically friends who are asthmatic as well, their attitudes towards it, a lot of them are a bit more laid back about it and don't fight it as much as what I do. They are quite happy to take all the drugs under the sun, which is fine if that's your attitude. I prefer to fight it.

> Her previous family doctor appeared to have contributed to this reasoning: Old Doctor H ... he was never one for giving you steroid inhalers unless it was absolutely necessary. I think it's just his attitudes wore off during the years. He's [current doctor] just a bit laid back about it all and he's quite happy just to fill you full of drugs. If you've got a problem, we'll give you something for it sort of thing. I prefer just to fight it more.

To fully accept the recommended regime also went against her upbringing, principally her father's fight against asthma. Accepting treatment required a loss of autonomy or a change in self-image that implied a failure or weakness on her part. Accepting treatment, especially long-term treatment that was perceived as powerful, required her to '*give in.*' More treatment implied greater illness, not better care.

> It's just the way my dad brought me up. 'Cause he lost his brother through asthma, so since then he's told everybody to fight it. I think it gives you more of a chance if you're willing to fight what you've got.

Intentions and actual medication use: This fight translated into a reluctance to use inhaled steroids and the long-acting inhaled beta-2-agonist, salmeterol, which she saw as the most powerful medicines. Although she was taking only half the recommended dose, she still perceived herself as taking them too often. Consequently she continually minimized the amount of these medications she consumed, despite the fact that she knew they improved her condition.

Jane demonstrated two unhelpful behaviors with her medicines, consuming twice the dose of the inhaled bronchodilator salbutamol (17 puffs/day) and less than half the dose of the steroid budesonide (1–2 puffs/day) recommended. In addition, she was on the oral contraceptive pill, which she took appropriately. She recognized that her family's experience with asthma had influenced her attitude.

> The Ventolin's there in case of an emergency so I don't panic, I know it's there. It's just basically the overall fight is against my asthma and not letting it win on top of me. I know my Ventolin's necessary, but sometimes you think there's always steroids if it's to be absolutely necessary. 'Cause I seen what they done to my dad and my sister, they're all huge.

Jane's coping strategy resulted from an understanding of both the condition and the treatment that was strongly based on her family's experiences and her perception that '*fighting it*' was more effective than using the treatment as advised. Although we cannot say what would have happened if her previous doctor had suggested the treatment, she clearly had insufficient trust in her current doctor to accept his opinion. She appears to be operating primarily according to her values rather than as a result of an explicit testing process or trust in her doctor. The consequence is overuse of one medicine and underuse of another.

Case example: Jim

Jim was a 42-year-old man with a passion for sports.

Illness representations: Jim sustained a bruise while canoeing that was preventing him from taking part in a number of other sports. His view of the injury indicated that its severity and likely duration were unlikely to be particularly problematic for him.

> I went to the family doctor because there was some chest problem that I was aware of but I didn't know what was causing it. I went to get a diagnosis. ... Now there's been several times when it's a 'virus' causing the problem but the doctor says 'I can give you a prescription for it.' My response is 'Well, what's going to happen if I don't take anything?' and [the doctor says] 'Oh ... it'll probably clear up.'

Values: Jim demonstrates a strong dislike of allopathic medicines – a view supported by his family network and illustrated by the fact that he had not had his children immunized. He consciously uses his doctor to exclude serious disease, and by implication he appears to have some trust in this relationship. However, he explicitly tests out his own approach while holding the prescribed therapy in reserve. In this instance, probably wisely, Jim declined to use a non-steroidal anti-inflammatory preparation, but happily took arnica, a homeopathic remedy, instead. His attitude to medication is clear from the following quote:

> Most of the drugs are new. They haven't been proven over a long period of time, so the more I can keep clear of them the happier I am. Not only does it mean I'm not taking a chemical with unknown side-effects, this is also actually boosting my body's immunity ... or I feel it is.

Intentions and actual medication use: Jim was reasonably pragmatic. His values largely favoured 'natural' remedies. However, he also recognized that where these did not work, prescribed medications might be necessary.

> So in that case I would take the prescription and wait for two or three days to see if it does clear up. And it always has. Because once I know what's wrong and I know it's not something serious, then I'm quite willing to say 'Well, my body can take care of itself', rather than ramming these drugs into it.

Route 3: the dominance of consulting and testing

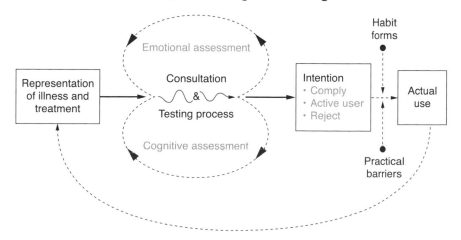

Figure 5.4 Route 3: the dominance of consulting and testing.

Case example: Joan

Joan was a 40-year-old woman who was living with her second husband in a large suburban estate. She had a daughter and a teenage son.

Illness representations: Joan had a long history of depression. When explaining her depression, she reported being taken into residential care during her childhood when her mother had herself suffered from severe depression. She thought that her mother's depression had led to her own, possibly through her '*genes*', but also through the unstable childhood that she had experienced. Her experience of being brought up by a mother with depression also informed her knowledge of what depression was and how bad it could be.

Joan reported that shortly after she married her first husband he started 'torturing' her. He beat her up and, knowing her fear of insects and spiders, started putting large spiders and '*creepy crawlies*' down her blouse. Her son then received a severe burn to his shoulder and had to attend a hospital for skin grafts. Joan felt that these family problems had combined to precipitate her illness. As her understanding of depression was so heavily based on past and present family experiences, she was particularly concerned for the welfare of her own children. She felt that unless she sought help, there was a strong chance that her children might also develop this terrible illness. This provided a very clear motivation for her to seek help and subsequently commence antidepressant treatment.

Consultation and testing: Joan knew that her mother had used antidepressants. However, she was also aware that these had not completely removed the depression, as her mother had eventually received a course of ECT. However, Joan was particularly concerned about being admitted to a psychiatric hospital and possibly having her children taken away from her. Consequently she accepted a prescription for antidepressants. She desperately wanted to feel better, and for this reason she took the tablets exactly as prescribed. However, after she had been taking the medication for 2 weeks she felt no better, and she began to worry that she was now going to be depressed for the rest of her life. She telephoned her family practitioner, who indicated that she should probably not expect to feel much different for at least 2 to 3 weeks, and suggested that she persist for a little longer. Joan decided to continue with the medication, and 10 days later began to feel that her mood had lifted. Her friends and family also began to comment that she both looked and sounded different.

Intention and actual medication use: Joan continued to take her medication religiously for over 2 years, with regular visits to her family practitioner. She developed a routine for her tablet taking, and accustomed herself to the possibility that she might need to continue the antidepressants indefinitely and felt that her '*life is built around them.*' Although Joan indicated that she would rather not have to take antidepressants, she was also very aware of how dreadful an experience she had been through when the depression was at its worst. She did not want to risk this recurring. She described her life as finally being stable, although she was constantly '*walking a fine line, a tightrope*' which she would fall off if she didn't take her medicine. It wouldn't simply be a matter of going through a few weeks of hell, but her life would gradually get worse and worse. Joan therefore had very strong feelings about not stopping her antidepressants in case this jeopardized her children's upbringing. She intended to continue taking her antidepressants indefinitely, and was nervous of her doctor suggesting any change. Her current routine was working for her and as such should not be changed.

Case example: Frank

Those on long-term treatments commonly consciously test out their therapy before accepting it. How it is tested depends on the patient's understanding of its function. For example, an analgesic with a short-term, symptomatic effect could be easily assessed whilst an anti-hypertensive may be stopped with no symptomatic consequences. Unless blood pressure measurement is understood and trusted such testing could be misinterpreted. Patients need to know how to assess a treatment's effect appropriately, otherwise they may select misleading measures or indicators. Frank's experience of starting clozapine, described below, illustrates some of these problems and uncertainties. It also demonstrates that in cases where the medicine is seen to be reducing symptoms, this can refocus attention on side-effects, which can then be seen as increasingly problematic. The testing process is not necessarily a 'one-off', but may be a continuous appraisal during which the key valued outcomes can change.

Illness representation: Frank was a 28-year-old man with a 6-year history of schizophrenia. Although he was clear what diagnosis he had been given, he continued to wonder whether it was in fact correct. He had previously been told that he had bipolar disorder, and before that major depression. He now maintained what he felt was a healthy scepticism about his current label of schizophrenia. Although he sometimes wondered about the title, he was much clearer in his own mind as to what constituted his illness. Most of the time he knew that his voices were part of his illness and he also knew that his low mood was part of it, too. However, he was sometimes confused as to whether other experiences such as slurred speech were to do with the illness or the treatment.

Consultation and testing: Over the past 2 years Frank had switched from one antipsychotic drug to another. However, all of those that he had tried had been relatively ineffective. Frank's consultant eventually suggested that he should try an atypical antipsychotic, clozapine. Frank also spoke to other staff members, his parents and other patients before deciding to try the drug.

After some time, Frank thought that the clozapine might be having an effect, but he was unsure about this. However, he was feeling extremely lethargic, and woke up each morning to find that he had been salivating excessively and needed to change his pillow. Prior to commencing clozapine he had been informed that there might be some initial side-effects and that there would be a delay in the benefits of the drug. However, the length of this delay was reported differently. Some people had said it would be around 6 months while others had said it could take up to 4 years. Frank decided to continue with the clozapine for at least 6 months to see whether it would work. He knew other people with schizophrenia who had given up after only a few weeks or months as their deadlines for improvement passed.

Intention and actual medication use: Frank described some significant side-effects on commencement of the drug, particularly debilitating drowsiness, but some people had said that he seemed better even though he didn't really feel it.

Over the next few months he reported that the drowsiness was becoming less problematic and the voices and visual hallucinations were diminishing. With some of the positive symptoms of schizophrenia diminishing, he developed new hope for the future. He could function better and think more clearly. He was full of praise for the drug, and he had developed a routine that he largely managed to maintain, so he intended to continue taking clozapine as long as it was working.

Values: As Frank's symptoms receded, his life changed and things that had not been a part of his life for many years became possible again. He started driving again, took a part-time job and started playing golf again. As the possibilities changed, new values became important. However, his new lifestyle and growing range of opportunities meant that his previously less problematic experiences came to be seen as limiting and as potential obstacles to a more 'normal' life.

> The only thing is the drooling in the pillow when I am sleeping. It doesn't bother me, but if I get a girlfriend that might bother her when that comes on …

As a result it was clear that the assessment process was repeated over time, with Frank repeatedly considering whether the drug was benefiting him or not. However, the criteria against which he judged the medicine changed as his life and social situation changed. Eventually he came to a point where he recognized that some of his remaining symptoms of schizophrenia could possibly be improved further through an increase in dose.

> I think I could feel better if I got more clozapine. If I got more clozapine I would be feeling better, but I couldnae be bothered going back into the hospital. So I'll just stick with what I am on because they would need to monitor it and take my blood pressure and all that.

The testing eventually fed back into his understanding of the treatment and through to his motivation to consider further changes in his medication.

Case examples in overview

From these case studies it is evident that there are both similarities and differences between individuals. Although three routes have been highlighted, the reality may be more complex, with elements of each playing a role at any one time, differing primarily in emphasis.

For most people, after an initial period of active consideration there is some degree of acceptance and integration of the drug into their life. There may be some ongoing monitoring of the way in which the medicine and its effects are impacting on the patient's life, and this may be intentional or subconscious. However, even if the drug is fully accepted in principle, the regimen may not be. Even with an adequate understanding of a drug, knowledge of prescription instructions and successful experience of following the treatment, some patients find that they cannot use medicines in an appropriate way. Whether people see themselves as passive *compliers* with the doctor's instructions or as being in control and modifying use to address their problems, they may still have practical difficulties successfully fitting this into their lives. Indeed, if these problems are sufficiently severe, they may force a change in treatment, modification of the regime, or a revisiting of the whole process.

A point is hopefully reached where there is an *intention*, for whatever reason, to use treatment in a particular way. It is at this point that practical issues may obstruct treatment or at times provide convenient excuses for patients' use of treatment to fall below that intended even by them. Obviously these can be genuine barriers, as suggested by the falling use of medicines with increasing frequency of dosing, a particular problem with the very demanding regimes for HIV. Other patients, such as clozapine users, have to attend regularly for monitoring, or have particular difficulties due to concentration or memory problems. However, it is also more socially acceptable to *forget* pills than to disagree with your clinician's advice. Patients who want to take a treatment will be able to read the label, seek guidance from a pharmacist or devise ways of prompting themselves if required. For example, Jane established various systems for her rapid need for salbutamol at any time. She kept numerous 'spares' at home and at work, and kept one in a pocket when she was working outdoors to prevent it from freezing up in winter. Her pattern of excessive salbutamol use and inadequate steroid use developed despite her partner regularly reminding her about the latter, so recall was not the problem. Indeed the participants in our interviews reported a wide range of solutions (*see* Table 5.1).

Table 5.1 Potential solutions to problems with taking medication

Problem	Solutions witnessed
Confusion	Reminder from partner/carer or use of dosing system (dosette or laying out medication)
Remembering to take medication	Tie with routine (e.g. bedtime or a meal) Assistance from carers or alarm clock
Knowing that one has taken medication	Laying out in advance (e.g. in egg cups) Device with days/times labelled
Running out of medication	Order in advance, keep a spare, mark on calendar
Frequency of administration	Not readily solved, especially if working
Side-effects	Modify dose or timing (e.g. diuretics and travel)

Once a treatment is accepted it becomes '*part of life*', built into the daily routine, and is no longer an issue. This can be demonstrated by people omitting to mention some long-standing therapies because they seem so trivial to them (e.g. the oral contraceptive pill).

Stability or fluidity in patients' use of medications

Medication use is not static. As Frank's story demonstrates, symptoms, knowledge, attitudes and values can change, leading people to review their own medication use. The cycle may be re-entered when new information or treatment requires evaluation. In Jane's case she perceived her situation to be acceptable, although her family doctor was known to be unhappy about her pattern of treatment use. There was little likelihood of her current doctor influencing her behavior, as she had little faith in his advice. Only when her interpretation of the nature of her problem changes or she understands her inhalers better might she 'fight' her disease by more effective use of her medicines. However, rather than telling her what to do, which can be seen to challenge her desire for control, perhaps she could be invited to conduct her own reappraisal. Perhaps she could be helped to convince herself.

The consultation in the wider healthcare context

From these cases it can be seen that the history of and story behind the illness have a very powerful influence on reasoning and on the types of responses that an individual might be willing to make to a perceived disease. The *popular sector* concept appears to be dominant. Although the decision to consult stems from their illness and treatment beliefs, it is clear from patients' accounts that consultations with clinicians can be very influential. Once patients elect to seek professional help, there is an opportunity to modify the way they see things – to reframe their illness beliefs. The TDM suggests that this can be done in both a cognitive manner, through information giving, and via the connection or relationship between the parties, on a more intuitive or emotive level. If the professional explanation fits well with their existing interpretation, they should easily combine to reinforce a strategy that is unlikely to be contentious. If there are substantive differences then it will require a high degree of trust in the clinician or very effective information-giving skills to bring the patient towards the view of the professional sector. For some people, the doctor's view simply cannot be reconciled with their own understanding of either their illness or the proposed treatments. This is drug specific, and may result in treatments being rejected and alternatives sought elsewhere. For instance, Jane accepted and indeed overused salbutamol, but rejected her preventive steroid, budesonide.

Conclusion

In summary, in this chapter we have sought to demonstrate that patients' stories and explanations about their illness experiences, including those with medications, are an effective way to understand their behaviors. Although accessing feelings, ideas and expectations has long been a mainstay of patient-centered medicine, we have sought to show how it is possible to use these in a focussed way with regard to medicines. Not only will exploring these areas enhance the connection or therapeutic relationship that is formed and allow the patient's perspective to be included more, but also it can provide invaluable insights into behavior, including medication use. For a listener who is familiar with behavioral models, it is possible to focus on what is driving unhelpful behaviors, which provides the opportunity for more considered interventions to modify these, if appropriate.

Picking up on the popular, professional and folk sectors of healthcare described in Chapter 2 and in particular the *therapeutic decision model*, we have sought to flesh these out with selected examples. We have shown how patients hold illness beliefs or '*representations*' about both their illness and their treatment that can be considered in terms of Leventhal's dimensions of identity, cause, consequences, time line and cure/control. In addition, we have illustrated how these beliefs have influenced help seeking, coping strategies and medication use in individual cases. These beliefs not only influence decisions directly, but also have a substantial effect on the cognitive testing process which, it was argued in Chapter 3, is a fundamental element of the journey of many patients through this process. If a patient expects a medicine to produce a specific effect within a specific time period, they are likely to be disappointed if this does not occur, and they may modify their use of the medication as a result. This process, in its various forms, is almost universal and forms the core of the TDM. Whether a deliberate test, accumulated observations or lack of achievement of an outcome, clinicians should recognize that a patient's interpretation of events will carry great weight. Unless patients' values dictate that they will not even try a treatment, every prescription can be regarded as an experiment for that individual. Of course common practice acknowledges this, and frequently patients are reviewed 'to see how you are getting along.' However, it is less common for patients' beliefs or expectations to be aired or incorporated within this process. As around half of the medicines prescribed are being taken reasonably well despite the apparently poor job we are doing at present, this may not be an efficient use of time on every occasion a prescription is issued. The point here is to illustrate how useful these accounts can be when required.

Finally, we have tried to place the practical barriers that are often cited as the reason for *non-compliance* in perspective at the end of a much larger process. The implication is that these can usually be overcome for patients who want to take their medicines optimally.

Using patients' stories, we have presented illustrative examples and have deliberately selected many of these from patients with severe and enduring mental health problems, the type of patient whose views are often discounted. Because of the nature of these research studies, it is likely that these patients were telling the truth, or as near to it as recall would allow, and this is obviously an important consideration. In most cases we were able to gather confirmation through pill counts, patient records or relatives – an option commonly available in practice. The climate in which these stories are accessed is critical, a point that is discussed in detail in Chapter 6, as the clinical environment may be quite different to that of a research interview.

Finding common ground

Jon Dowell

The secret of the care of the patient is in caring for the patient.

(Peabody, 1984)

In Chapter 1 it was established that around one-third of people in the western world receive long-term medication, about half of whom do not use it as prescribed. This is believed to be responsible for considerable ill health and death. The complexities of medication use as a form of human behavior have been discussed in Chapters 2, 3 and 4 with reference to evidence of what happens to medicines, so-called lay models of health and remedies, as well as many of the psychological models that have been applied to this topic. In Chapter 5 we presented a schematic *therapeutic decision model* designed to assimilate the key elements into a comprehensive framework that can inform clinicians considering individual patients. This emphasizes that patients are commonly active problem solvers, making initial decisions based on their underlying values and beliefs, although often in the context of a therapeutic clinical relationship of some kind. Preliminary decisions are then informed by their evaluation of treatment, both cognitive and emotional, which should be seen as a core component of the decision-making process. The next two chapters will translate these conceptual ideas into a consultation method, borrowing from the emerging literature on so-called shared decision making and our own research into managing known *non-compliance* using these techniques. Of course resolving inconsistencies for individuals in this process is bound to be an inexact process – more of an art or craft than a science. The approach described remains open to local interpretation, and artistic licence should be used. To quote from Neighbour's book, *The Inner Consultation*:

> As you know, practising medicine can be exhilarating. But to become a little more skilful does mean extending your repertoire of professional behaviour and trying things the results of which you can initially only imagine. The price of exhilaration is risk. To live safely with risk you need a degree of trust and commitment.
>
> (Neighbour, 1987)

The remainder of the book is therefore aimed directly at prescribers – at *you* as a clinician. In order to refine your consulting skills you will need to take risks and try out the techniques we describe, otherwise your repertoire will not extend. Hopefully the case studies and quotes will provide sufficiently convincing evidence for you to think it is worth having a go, and to trust this text and your own therapeutic relationships with patients. These chapters do not aim to tell you how to do it, but rather to indicate the things you should consider while you try. We include some of the phrases and aids that we found helpful as a starting point, but you will want to modify these according to your own style.

The 'normal' and the 'special' situation

For practical purposes it can be helpful to classify and consider patient-centered prescribing in terms of two types of interaction. In the 'normal' consultation there would be no reason for expecting substantive discordance between the views of the clinician and the patient. When experience suggests, or there are other reasons for suspecting that divergent views are present, the consultation may be considered 'special', to varying degrees. The 'normal' situation would be typified by a consultation with a clearly competent patient with a similar cultural background to the clinician and no significant complicating psychological factors. Here it might be expected that common ground will be easily found and quickly acknowledged by both parties. These interactions follow predictable patterns, are highly efficient, and represent what might be seen as day-to-day practice. This is a simple extension of what Stewart and colleagues have termed '*finding common ground*', and will be considered in this chapter. In addition, some other recent models of shared decision making will be discussed here, along with their potential difficulties, the need to balance likely benefits with available resources, and how other professionals may assist the process.

However, there are also instances when clinicians can anticipate problems or they become aware of them and would ideally modify their approach in order to manage them (Gwyn and Elwyn, 1999). For instance, computerized systems increasingly alert us to *non-compliance*. Alternatively, empowered patients are increasingly vocalising their views and preferences before the clinician does so. Sometimes these may clearly stem from cultural origins, but they may also reflect fear of medicines or a positive stance towards particular therapies, and not necessarily different cultural perspectives. These occasions present different challenges that may merit investing additional time and specific techniques if frustrating impasses are to be avoided. These 'special' situations are considered in depth in Chapter 7, where techniques for diagnosing problems and suggested solutions are offered.

Common ground under 'normal' conditions

From different stables subtly different approaches have arisen to essentially the same issue, namely agreeing on common goals and approaches to managing medical problems with patients. We see no substantive conflict between 'finding common ground', 'shared decision making' and 'concordance', which are all ways of achieving patient-centered prescribing. Whatever label or approach is applied, the task must surely involve elucidating the patient's perspective on their situation and options, which itself requires a suitable climate for patients to feel able to openly discuss their views and allow the clinician to explore and potentially challenge them. Patient-centered prescribing requires the clinician to believe that this is the preferable way to provide care, and that it is morally correct, rather than a way of creating *compliance*, as patients may make decisions with which the clinician disagrees. If the clinician or medical convention assumes precedence over the patient's values, then they may be deterred from being open, their autonomy may be compromised and the opportunity for therapeutic partnership may be lost.

There is emerging evidence that patient care improves when choices are genuinely offered (so far primarily in terms of satisfaction), but at present there is only tentative evidence that health outcomes improve, and it must be recognized that this is to some extent a leap of faith. But then who is to judge whether living a little longer is preferable to living with a side-effect (e.g. impotence caused by a beta-blocker)? Or whether glycaemic control is the most important consideration for an unhappy and resentful youngster who has learned to hate their insulin injections? Patient-centered prescribing must be judged by patient-centered outcome measures, and valid ones are not yet available.

There is a real danger that this process may become a sophisticated way of manipulating patients gently towards the 'medical view' unless there is a genuine willingness to let them express their preferences and make their own choices. The anxieties that clinicians may feel as a result are discussed in Chapter 8, but the danger of manipulation must be considered before attention is given to the components of any decision-sharing process.

Atmosphere and trust

It is extremely difficult to know what impact one is having in any human interaction, and it is often impossible or inappropriate to ask explicitly. This is part of the craft of clinical communication. Although further research would be helpful in this area, we already know that the non-verbal components of the interaction are likely to be most revealing in this regard (Silverman *et al.*, 1998). Some patients will feel at ease immediately, but many will not. This is a particular problem if, for whatever reason, the patient feels that their preferences, behavior or use of treatment may induce disapproval. Powerful traditions have evolved to govern acceptable roles within medical encounters that are extremely useful because they enable intimate information to be exchanged and physical examinations to be performed. However, there is also a substantive imbalance in power that still underlies most interactions. As a result, many patients find it difficult to openly discuss the way in which they use or wish to use treatment for fear of courting criticism, jeopardising the clinical relationship or perhaps implying criticism of the prescriber. An analysis by Barry *et al.* (2000) of 35 consultations and associated patient interviews found that unvoiced agenda items were part of the problem in all 14 interactions with a 'problem outcome.' Consequently, clinicians who commence consultations with a traditional style, even if they are genuinely willing and able to change, will have begun by reinforcing the prevailing model, and may have made their patient less likely to openly discuss their situation. The context and initial tone of the encounter should ideally encourage patients – indeed empower them – to contribute their views openly as well as their planned or actual behavior. Token statements such as 'I know many people find taking their tablets every day difficult' are inadequate. It is important to avoid such accusations until a sufficiently trusting climate has been established. Then apparently quite challenging statements may be more acceptable and may generate constructive exchanges. The subtlety of this process is indicated in an intriguing study by Ambady *et al.* (2002), who found that surgeons' tone of voice as assessed from just four 10-second audio clips (in terms of warmth, hostility, dominance and anxiety) significantly reflected their malpractice claims history. In addition, Mercer *et al.* (2002) reported that perceived empathy, as rated by patients, was the single most important factor enhancing so-called 'enablement' in a series of 200 consultations at the Glasgow Homeopathic Hospital. It seems that non-verbal components may be a critical factor here, in addition to the content of the clinician's talk. Hence it is probably more important to believe in the approach than to seek to master the skills, as these may not come across as genuine.

Case example: Rebecca

Rebecca was an epileptic woman with suspected poor compliance. She resented her disease and medication, and felt that treatment made her feel unwell after some months, although she knew that it suppressed her seizures. She had developed a strategy of not taking her medicine for about 3 months at a time, and felt that she knew her condition well enough to know when to resume her medicine in order to prevent further seizures. She would then restart her medication and continue it for 6 to 9 months. She had been seizure free for 2 years, felt that she had control over her condition, and did not want further intervention or drug changes. Here she first describes how she 'hates' having fits, and then discloses her non-compliance.

> Rebecca: *"The last one I had it was in the evening, which was ... I didn't like it because I wet myself. I'd never wet myself before. I was sick and it was a long time since I've been sick. I just hated it. I was absolutely 'Oh not doing this again.' Panic. I just hated it."*
>
> Rebecca: *"Well, I was on phenytoin before I got changed on to the new ones. I was taking six of them, which is a lot to take in one day."*
> Dr Albert: *"It's a nightmare, isn't it?"*
> Rebecca: *"And I was on the pill and I could have had about half a dozen children because this wasn't very good. No, since I got changed to the other ones."*
> Dr Albert: *"So you're happier. The medicines you're taking now you're much happier with?"*
> Rebecca: *"Yes."*
> Dr Albert: *"How long ago was that change made?"*
> Rebecca: *"Trying to think ... about two years ... three years. Something like that."*
> Dr Albert: *"How about these ones?"*
> Rebecca: *"Oh, I do sometimes not take them. Sometimes I do get fed up taking tablets. Does that sound ...? That sounds daft."*
> Dr Albert: *"No, it doesn't sound daft. No, no. I can completely sympathise with that. I think that it's really hard sometimes having to take these things all the time."*
> Rebecca: *"Yeah. It is."*

This doctor's empathic responses allowed the patient to begin to discuss her *non-compliance*. However, perhaps more importantly, the patient's behavior and feelings with regard to her treatment are also being welcomed, not dismissed. By valuing these experiences, the possibility of this patient having a significant influence on future treatment decisions is being created. However, there is a fine line to tread between creating a therapeutic relationship that is used to inform and help a patient, and creating one that is used to pressure them into agreeing to the clinician's suggestions.

This theme will be revisited in Chapter 8, when the delicate issue of being seen to allow patients to reject treatment is discussed.

On a more positive note, the trusting nature of many if not most doctor–patient relationships (as indicated in the *therapeutic decision model*) is an important reason why as much as 50–60% of medicines are taken at all. Valuing and developing trusting clinical relationships is a key component of all consultation models, for good reason. Not only will it encourage open information exchange, but it will also facilitate all forms of decision making.

Finding common ground

Interest in patient involvement in the decision-making process is not new, and Tuckett's seminal study in the early 1980s reported only 22 examples of patient involvement in therapeutic decisions from over 2000 general practice consultations in the UK (Tuckett *et al.*, 1985). More recent studies suggest that this situation has changed little despite a widespread shift towards patient participation, partnership and autonomy (Stevenson *et al.*, 2000; Campion *et al.*, 2002). As it appears that this process is difficult to achieve, let us now consider the process of involving patients in decisions more closely when this is deemed to be required in relatively straightforward situations. The more challenging situations are discussed in Chapter 7.

There are a number of models of shared decision making that are worth considering briefly, primarily to illustrate the extent to which they overlap. Stewart and colleagues were the first to explicate different elements in the process which they termed *finding common ground*. In *Patient-Centered Medicine: Transforming the Clinical Method* (Stewart *et al.*, 1995), this later element of the consultation process was described relatively briefly, reflecting how novel exploring the illness experience was considered to be at that time, and illustrating how far shared decision making has evolved since. However, in their more recent text and indeed in others this element of patient-centered care has expanded considerably (Edwards and Elwyn, 2002; Stewart *et al.*, 2003). Reaching agreement about the goals of treatment, the choice of treatment and actions to be taken is now depicted as a far more central element of the interaction, and is also described in more detail (Stewart *et al.*, 1995, 2003).

Stewart and colleagues describe four elements in the process that they call '*finding common ground*', and others have produced comparable analyses, which we shall also outline here.

Finding common ground involves the following processes.

- **Defining the problem.** Before trying to decide on the response, it is essential to establish a shared view of the problem. Is it possible to agree what the illness represents? Is a sore throat a self-limiting viral illness or the harbinger of rheumatic fever or quinsy?
- **Defining the goals.** What do the respective parties expect or want to achieve? Does the patient feel that they need antibiotics while the clinician seeks to avoid 'irrational' prescribing and modify future help-seeking behavior? Clearly it is difficult to achieve a mutually satisfactory solution with such divergent goals. Divergence is likely to prove emotive for both parties, and clinicians should be able to recognize and deal with this through discussion, which might include being able to say 'no' effectively if necessary.

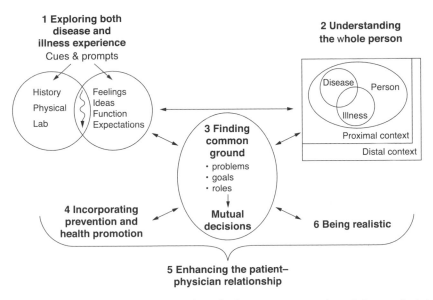

Figure 6.1 The patient-centered clinical method. Patient-centered medicine as depicted by Stewart *et al.* (2003). Reproduced with the permission of the copyright holder.

- **Defining the roles of doctor and patient.** This might include a pragmatic distribution of tasks or responsibilities (medicine taking, arranging investigations or making a referral) to help to summarize and close an interaction or become a key element when the clinician and the patient are in 'profound disagreement.' If the relationship is failing to function effectively, it can help to re-establish the fundamentals – a repair manoeuvre.
- **The process of finding common ground.** This is portrayed as being led by the professional, who lays out their 'definition' of the above components and then helps the patient to raise questions, concerns and issues that might alter the plan. It is suggested that clinicians have a duty to be flexible in the event of disagreement, but that this can be managed by showing respect while at the same time being explicit about the issues involved.

However, more structured guidance on how shared decisions can be achieved has been offered by others (Towle and Godolphin, 1999; Edwards and Elwyn, 2002), and this is part of a growing literature describing the ideal decision-making process that, it is suggested, should be discernible during most interactions. With their strong rational or cognitive focus, these approaches seem to err more towards evidence-based practice than patient-centered approaches, but can be seen as part of a toolkit that can help practitioners to vary their approach according to the situation and patient need.

Other models of shared decision making (SDM)

What would happen if 'We have some choices and they are ...' was in the doctor's habitual script and 'What's the evidence for that, doctor?' was in the patient's?

(Godolphin, 2003)

Edwards and Elwyn present a detailed analysis of the decision-making process, including a more conceptual analysis of the possible range, from the paternalistic 'doctor knows best' to informed patient choice (Edwards and Elwyn, 2002). Within this they highlight three key components, namely *information exchange, deliberation* and the *agency* (or ownership) of the decision itself. These differ, so that, for instance, in a 'paternalistic' framework the professional makes the decision on the patient's behalf, whereas in the 'informed' mode the patient makes their own decision without the clinician's input. From this point Edwards and Elwyn argue that the more holistic approach (as epitomized by the description by Stewart and colleagues) can be usefully married with a more task-orientated one. The knack is to recognize that the whole interaction consists of more than its constituent parts, and that the 'practical wisdom' or 'right brain' contribution should be seen as essential.

On the basis of a study in which groups of family doctors deconstructed the process of sharing decisions to identify the constituent parts, Elwyn and colleagues conclude that there are nine distinct components. However, they highlight the fact that these can occur within a broader interaction, and need not occur sequentially as they are presented on paper (Elwyn *et al.,* 2000).

These components may be summarized as follows.

1 Involve the patient in the decision process (implicit or explicitly).
2 Define and agree about the problem.
3 Explore ideas, fears and expectations with regard to the problem/treatments.
4 Portray the options.
5 Elicit format preferences and provide tailored information.
6 Check understanding and reactions.
7 Check whether the patient accepts the process and their role in it.
8 Make, discuss or defer the decision.
9 Agree action and follow-up.

A number of explicit additional tasks are introduced here – for instance, assessing preferences for information provision and role in the decision-making process. Likewise, the clinician's duty to portray the choices available implies a far greater attention to detail. These skills are described in more depth in *Evidence-Based Patient Choice* (Edwards and Elwyn, 2002).

Towle and Godolphin (1999) defined a similar set of eight competencies for physicians using a process of literature review, interviews, and focus groups with both clinicians and patients. They explicitly suggest that clinicians should also access relevant evidence to inform their information provision.

These competencies are outlined as follows.

1 Develop a partnership with the patient.
2 Establish or review the patient's preferences for information (e.g. amount or format).
3 Establish or review the patient's preferences with regard to their role in decision making (e.g. risk taking and degree of involvement of self and others) and the existence and nature of any uncertainty about the course of action to take.
4 Ascertain and respond to the patient's ideas, concerns and expectations (e.g. about disease management options).
5 Identify choices (including ideas and information that the patient may have) and evaluate the research evidence in relation to the individual patient.

6 Present (or direct the patient to) the evidence, taking into account competencies 2 and 3, framing effects (how presentation of the information may influence decision making), etc. Help the patient to reflect on and assess the impact of alternative decisions with regard to his or her values and lifestyle.

7 Make or negotiate a decision in partnership with the patient, and resolve conflict.

8 Agree an action plan and complete arrangements for follow-up.

It is difficult to argue that any of these components in any of these models are not potentially useful, although precisely how the individual tasks are to be achieved, how a clinician can judge whether this has been done adequately, and the detail of resolving conflict remain sketchy. Both skill sets were derived through discussion about the process rather than observation of it in practice, so it remains to be seen whether they prove applicable or effective. They are currently being incorporated into communication skills texts, and training programmes and studies are beginning to assess their introduction (Silverman *et al.*, 1998; Elwyn *et al.*, 2001; Dowell *et al.*, 2004).

In addition to physician competencies, Towle and Godolphin also highlight the need for patients to have certain abilities in order to engage in this process. It is not known how widely these are held and, as many clinicians may suspect, it is not known to what extent this type of involvement is really wanted or likely to be beneficial (Coulter, 1999).

Case example: Terrance

Accepting illness and long-term treatment is something most people would wish to avoid, and some try to do so. Terrance was 54 years old when he was first told his blood pressure was high at a Well Man check, and he was asked to return for the measurement to be repeated. Although he is a biomedical laboratory scientist, he deliberately avoided returning until this was noticed 3 years later during his next visit to a doctor for an unrelated reason.

Illness representation: Terrance had avoided addressing this problem or considering its implications, although he could identify no special reason for this. However, the problem was fairly easy to ignore, as he had no symptoms that he attributed to high blood pressure, and he was not disabled by the condition in any way. He regarded himself as a fit man who did not want to acknowledge a diagnosis that seemed to highlight the ageing process.

Consultation and testing: When Terrance's dislike of having his blood pressure measured was remarked upon, his reluctance to be given this diagnosis became apparent. He simply did not wish to '*feel ill.*' Acknowledging his intellectual capacity, he was introduced to a cardiovascular risk calculator (which indicates the 10-year risk of stroke or ischaemic heart disease) and shown the implications of continuing to ignore his problem. Aware of the fact that Terrance had previously avoided repeat measurements, his doctor emphasized the role of measurement error as well as the fact that he could decide about treatment if the diagnosis was confirmed. He was left with an informed decision to make and given a meter to assess his blood pressure at home as a means of convincing him of the diagnosis rather than identifying any potential 'white-coat' effect.

Intention and actual medication use: Terrance did return, and once it had been demonstrated that reduced salt intake had not resolved the problem, he elected to receive treatment, which he now monitors himself at home.

If we accept that more informed decision sharing like that described above is desirable but rarely practiced, we must also accept that it will require some additional time to meaningfully achieve these tasks and to begin to consider when this investment is likely to be worthwhile. There is an 'opportunity cost' to be considered and balanced against the considerable costs of suboptimal healthcare if effective treatments are not used because patients are not brought into the process successfully. At this point it is necessary to introduce some additional factors that make decision making particularly difficult to understand, and sometimes bewildering. These are doubts about rationality and doubts about information provision.

Doubts about rationality

Even in studies where considerable efforts have been made to achieve sufficient understanding about risks, a proportion of patients make choices that appear illogical and differ from doctors' views. For instance, 50% of patients with atrial fibrillation would accept substantive risks of major bleeds from anticoagulation therapy in order to obtain a minimal reduction in the risk of stroke (Devereaux *et al.*, 2002). Across a broader range of conditions, Montgomery and Fahey (2001) report that patients' choices about treatment are often not congruent with doctors' interpretation of even the best available evidence. Thus even under research conditions, where additional time and communication aids are available, patients' choices often do not match evidence-based recommendations or clinicians' views. At present the reasons for this can only be guessed at, but the implication is that discordance between patient choice and clinicians' recommendations is a common event. Disentangling whether the communication has failed to successfully convey the risks and benefits or whether patients are applying different value systems is a perpetual problem.

Doubts about information provision

There is currently insufficient understanding about information transfer in the clinical setting, and no common language of risk that allows us to provide relevant information in a way that will be reliably understood (Coulter *et al.*, 1999; Paling, 2003). Even without major cultural or linguistic barriers, it is clear that the presentation of risk (numerically, graphically and verbally framing data) has an effect on the choices that are made (Gigerenzer, 2002; Edwards *et al.*, 2003a). It has been suggested that the degree of trust in the source, the relationship to other perceived risks, the fit with previous knowledge and experience, and the relevance for everyday life, as well as the difficulty and importance of the decision, all influence how information is assimilated (Alaszewski and Horlick-Jones, 2003). No clinician can thoroughly assess and address all of these issues in routine practice, so feasible ways of focussing on the key influential components for the individual in question must be found. However, even this requires care, as attempts to provide information in an effective way may easily lead to its manipulation in order to induce the decision that the clinician favours (Gigerenzer and Edwards, 2003). A 'sensible choice' can itself be interpreted as confirmation that the information was indeed understood precisely because it led to the obvious choice. So clinicians have the difficult task of conveying information and checking that it has been understood without using an apparently rational choice as the marker of this. Otherwise they risk altering the way in which they present information and manipulating the decision until their favoured conclusion is reached.

Feasibility

Although it has been demonstrated that patient-centered consultation can be more effective and take no longer than the more traditional history-taking approach, this has not yet been shown for the closing half of the interaction. Descriptions of 'shared decision making' have been largely theoretically derived, their use is not yet common, and there may be reasons for this.

In order to study more precisely how shared decisions are made in practice, Robertson recently performed an analysis of the discourse from 30 consultations which patients rated very highly for their involvement in the treatment decisions (using the COMRADE questionnaire; Edwards *et al.*, 2003b). Despite these being reportedly exemplary illustrations of shared decisions, there were only four examples of patients being explicitly involved out of 59 decisions (Robertson, 2004). The only actual decision left to a patient was whether to be referred to specialists via the National Health Service or privately. Thus it appears to be possible, under normal general practice conditions, for patients to feel adequately involved even if they have not been formally involved as recent authors suggest that they should. Elwyn *et al.* (2001) reported similar findings. A 'sense' of partnership appears to obviate the need for much of the detail, and during 'normal' consultations it may be acceptable and efficient to use this (at least in the UK, where patients are often cognisant of time pressures) (Cromarty, 1996). In addition, a number of qualitative studies imply that patients can only make long-term decisions about medications once they know how they will be affected by them (Dowell *et al.*, 1996; Benson and Britten, 2002). Thus a relatively straightforward approach to an initial decision to simply try out a treatment may be an efficient way to practice when sufficient common ground can be established. This does not mean that the patient's ideas, concerns and expectations are not important, but that once these have been elicited it may often be safe for the clinician to make a recommendation to be tried out without needing to lay out the range of options available. Although this approach does risk perpetuating some of the existing unsatisfactory patterns of medication use, it is time efficient and allows patients to try out their treatment and therefore become more informed about it. Being realistic has always been a component of practicing patient-centered medicine, and here this may be represented by swift decisions about the extent to which clinician and patient are 'speaking the same language', or have 'connected' (Neighbour, 1987). If this appears to be adequate, one strategy would be to agree on a trial of treatment and to set parameters for the review, rather than engage in a detailed process of decision sharing that is wasted because a side-effect arises that dictates events. Creating the climate of partnership may be much more important than the formalities of sharing decisions. To extend Godolphin's argument:

> What would happen if 'These are the treatment options available for your blood pressure. Try each of them for a month and record how they affect you. Then we can discuss what would be best for you' was in the doctor's habitual script?

However, more structured approaches may be necessary when discordance is suspected, and indeed it seems sensible to focus resources on those occasions when investing additional time and effort is most likely to have an impact. Probably the most common marker of discordance is so-called *non-compliance*, particularly if it appears that clinical care is suboptimal as a result. Other examples include divergent beliefs about the disease or illness course, or a substantive cultural divide between clinician and patient. Of course, in order to assess these components it is necessary to have explored the patient's beliefs about their illness and the potential treatments in the first place. So a key component of the patient-centered approach provides critical insight into the need for a more formal decision-sharing process as well as information that is useful for doing so.

Purpose

Before leaving the notion of shared decision making on a pessimistic note, we must reflect on the broader picture. Although research seeks to understand the different components of shared decision making and the way in which these interact, often finding failings in both theory and practice as new knowledge emerges, we must not lose sight of the goal. Imperfect as our skills and working conditions are, there is no substantive voice arguing against patients being offered a greater role in their health-care decisions. There can be no doubt that a substantial proportion of patients wish to engage in this process, even if it is not for everyone all of the time. Therefore clinicians will be increasingly expected to share decisions to the best of their ability, and we should equip ourselves to do so, even in the knowledge that we clearly have a lot to learn about the process.

Although structured approaches enable us to understand and analyse what we do in practice and rehearse new skills, they can and will only be of use if we believe in the value of employing patient-centered approaches to the therapeutic decision. There may be a fundamental need for clinicians to consider their views on patient autonomy – no amount of skills training can alter how therapeutic decisions are approached. It is only possible to really enter into the 'mutual decision-making' element of patient-centered medicine when clinicians are willing to let patients make what they consider to be the wrong choices without attempting to talk them round. This reflects a mindset, not a skill, and is discussed further in Chapter 8, where we consider some of the challenging situations that can arise as a result of this process.

The role of other healthcare providers

We have been at pains to recognize that the act of prescribing is increasingly performed by pharmacists and nurses as well as doctors, and we would reinforce this again here. Roles are changing, and nurses especially are now making primary diagnostic decisions or changing treatments according to treatment protocols. Although there may be an increased expectation that these so-called 'supplementary' prescribers will adhere to guidelines or protocols, the issues are little different to those for all prescribers, and this whole text applies to them. Inflexible treatment algorithms will at times clash with patient-centered care, and this needs to be recognized and responded to, even if the response is to pass the decision on.

We are considering here how professionals other than the principal prescriber may play a part in the process. We have surely established by now that the act of taking a medicine lies at the end of an often emotive and complex process that can involve many people, not just the prescriber and the patient. But what of the clinicians, from any discipline, who find themselves involved in helping patients to decide how or even whether to use their treatments? Often this might involve nurses, pharmacists, dietitians, etc. (or other doctors who were not involved in the original decision), and all professionals have the potential to influence patients and should be mindful of the impact that their guidance might have.

Bajcar (2006) describes a model of the medication-taking process which has three modes that accord closely with the TDM presented in Chapter 5. These are *non-problematic*, *problematic* and *stunned*. The *problematic* mode is akin to the decision-making cycle of the TDM and, in Bajcar's view, arises when patients cannot make sense of their situation. Typically Bajcar found that conflicting information from different sources produced this state, and a contradictory account from different professionals is one such cause. Thus it is important for everyone to have a basic grasp of their potential to assist appropriate choices as well as to create doubt and indecision. This potential derives from two sources – empowerment and education.

Empowerment

It is well known that the power differential within the typical clinical encounter favours the clinician. One effect of this is that patients may shy away from presenting their view, asking questions or revealing their 'ignorance.' This unhelpful state of affairs can be improved by other professionals, not only by explaining and educating, but by empowering patients to consider their view as important and their concerns as legitimate. Patients can be prompted and assisted to raise issues through discussion or making a list to present at their next visit. Indeed there is some suggestion that such preparation prior to a clinic visit has measurable effects on disease control (Kaplan *et al.*, 1989). Professionals such as nurses and pharmacists can have a crucial bridging role, providing an opportunity for patients' concerns and doubts to be formulated and expressed. The value of this should be recognized and used explicitly.

Education

There are many reasons why a wide range of professionals might become involved in educating patients about their treatments. Commonly the normal dispensing processes require pharmacists or their staff to do this. Often chronic disease management protocols contain some element of medication monitoring (e.g. use or side-effects) and specific education (e.g. about inhaler techniques). In addition, there are frequent occasions within clinics or other encounters when treatments are discussed and opportunities arise to enhance understanding of the condition or treatment in ways that resolve contradictions or inconsistencies and allow patients to make sense of things. In this context, education can helpfully be seen as creating meaning rather than as conveying information, and increased approachability may also assist this.

Specifically it is likely that there will be opportunities to do the following.

- Review how a patient is getting along. This might involve exploring whether the treatment seems to be working or not. How can they tell? Are there any perceived side-effects? The resulting discussion provides an opportunity to develop understanding about treatment that includes the experiences of the patient (e.g. that

inhaled steroids take time to work and should not be judged in the same way as bronchodilators).
- Explore specific aspects of use. Recall, timing, techniques and managing trips away from home, etc. can all be important and also provide helpful information. For instance, so-called 'drug holidays' over weekends or longer periods are a recognized form of experimentation. It may be deliberately considered variation rather than ill-informed or forgetful use that is the issue (e.g. omitting potent diuretics prior to going shopping). However, experienced professionals can also offer essential tips and tricks that help patients to gain maximum benefit from their treatments when required.
- Explain the prescriber's perspective. Patients can easily misunderstand not only the illness or treatment but also the stance of the prescriber. This can be extremely difficult for the prescriber to address, even if they know about it, and especially if there is any suspicion about motives. For instance, there may be suspicions about financial factors (Dowell *et al.*, 1996). These types of issues are commonly presented as off-the-cuff remarks, and whether true or not they merit discussion. A third party is well positioned to resolve them most effectively if they are untrue. If they are true, the patient deserves to know.

It should be clear that there are valuable and varied roles through which all healthcare professionals can support the process of patient-centered prescribing. To do this, they need to be aware of typical patterns of medication use and the range of routes by which these may be arrived at. They have unique potential to assist, because they may be seen as more approachable than the clinician who prescribed the medication, and can offer further patient-centered support. This implies optimising decisions and medication use, not simply telling patients 'to comply' or sending them back to the prescriber. If this appears to present some associated risks, that is because it does. These risks are discussed in Chapter 8.

Conclusion

In Chapter 6 the importance of creating a conducive atmosphere within the consultation has been discussed alongside the more mechanistic components of sharing decisions. The pressures on all healthcare systems mean that we need to capitalize on the skills that practitioners develop for rapidly establishing effective therapeutic relationships, and to use these to ensure that there is sufficient patient involvement and commitment to decisions. However, patients vary in the extent to which they wish to participate, and clinicians should be able to adapt accordingly and provide explicit decision sharing when required. There are a number of models available to help them to achieve this, all of which have a similar content. All of the models emphasize the need for an underlying partnership, but none of them describe in detail how to address persistent disagreement. Other healthcare professionals often become aware of problems before the primary prescriber, and the contribution that they can make to supporting and sustaining considered decisions has also been discussed. Chapter 7 builds upon the above principles by considering how decisions can be opened up and reconsidered constructively in what we have termed 'special' situations, such as harmful medication use.

Finding common ground
in 'special' situations

Jon Dowell

This chapter presents a consultation model that has been derived to help clinicians to engage with patients with regard to medication use under what we have been considering as 'special' circumstances. It seeks to provide a practical approach, based on both sound theory and practical experience, which can be employed when difficulties are encountered or anticipated. The aim is to enable clinicians to approach the situation positively with a considered plan of action and some solutions to the problems that they may encounter.

We shall briefly describe the process by which this approach was derived before presenting a diagrammatic summary and discussing its application in practice. We shall then outline four cases that illustrate each of the four common issues encountered. This should equip you to experiment with developing your own ways of exploring these issues with your patients.

What is a 'special' situation?

What might trigger you to think it worth engaging in this more detailed and potentially more time-consuming approach? Clinicians have to be realistic about what they can achieve, and they need to make choices about how to use their time to best effect. Therefore it is important to be able to identify when to invest their time and energy with reasonable hope of gain. Clearly there is a spectrum here ranging from accidentally omitting therapy through conscious variations in medication use to the grossly atypical approaches to illness and treatments that those with personality disorders or severe mental illness might demonstrate. This chapter will focus on what we might see as the middle ground, and specifically does not advocate these techniques for the latter two groups. The reasons for this are discussed later. However, it does offer a strategy to use when patients appear to 'block', when suboptimal medication use is affecting care, or when a sense of frustration or loss of 'connection' occurs.

The first four chapters sought to explain how patients' understanding or belief systems could lead them to manage their illness in a way that conventional medicine would view as suboptimal. Examples would include those asthmatics, hypertensives and diabetics who manage their conditions by using long-term treatments on a symptomatic basis. They might also include those who decline to take treatments or stop them too early (e.g. patients who are prescribed antidepressants). Without wanting to discuss potential reasons, which we shall consider shortly, it is immediately obvious that patients' actions will depend upon their views not only of their illness but also of the treatments on offer. As a result, interactions with such patients can very easily become dysfunctional. For instance, one young asthmatic explained at interview how he always requested and collected his steroid inhaler because he knew that this prevented him 'getting a lecture' from the nurse at his asthma review.

Most commonly the need to seek a stronger therapeutic alliance occurs when the patient reveals suboptimal medication use or this becomes apparent through another route – perhaps the clinical records indicate that medication use cannot be effective, or a stash of unused medicines is found. Essentially, so-called *non-compliance* is encountered. Another occasion when the need for deeper engagement becomes apparent is when the subtle vibes, non-verbal cues or indeed expressed views reveal that there is a discordance of opinions. A common example of this is antibiotic prescribing. Here there is clear evidence that doctors and patients often fail to understand each other's perspectives, which results in many unnecessary prescriptions, and others being discontinued too early (Macfarlane *et al.*, 1997). So this approach need not purely be a response to *non-compliance* – it may also be used to prevent suboptimal use in the first place.

However, this is not a panacea, and we must acknowledge and highlight the fact that exploring either cognitive or emotive responses to illness and treatment is not always straightforward or necessarily effective. For instance, cognitive impairment for any reason will limit this, as potentially will personality disorders or major mental illness. Again a degree of realism must be brought to bear on this, especially when initially experimenting with these techniques. It is not wise to start with your 'heartsink' patients or other extreme challenges!

Part 1: The therapeutic alliance model

Most of the remainder of this chapter is based on a study that sought ways to understand and manage patients' suboptimal use of treatment within the setting of general practice in the UK (Dowell *et al.*, 2002). Specifically this study aimed to develop an effective strategy for discussing medication use within the consultation, exploring insights into why suboptimal use was occurring, and to establish a more constructive or concordant way forward.

Employing a modified action research approach, we used cycles of qualitative data collection and analysis alongside our clinical care (Whyte, 1991). Each round of consultations and analysis was used to inform, test and refine the approach as it developed. Three family doctors who were familiar with the *therapeutic decision model* (Dowell and Hudson, 1997), *concordance* (Blenkinsopp *et al.*, 1997) and the *patient-centered clinical method* (Stewart *et al.*, 1995) purposefully sought non-compliant adult patients. A total of 24 patients with conditions that included hypertension, asthma, hypercholesterolemia, diabetes and epilepsy were recruited. All of them had documented prescription requests at least 50% above or below the prescribed level, and poor clinical control of their condition. Therefore they were all known to be both non-compliant with their treatment regimes and suffering suboptimal care as a result (as judged from the clinician's perspective).

When recruiting patients, up to four extended consultations ('additional medical time to discuss their care in more detail') were offered, the importance of their perspective was made explicit, and it was emphasized that their values had precedence over the doctor's when negotiating decisions. Thus these consultations were unusual because of their length (25 minutes), research nature (they were audio-taped) and the need for a consent process. At least 3 months after the last consultation, patient opinion, clinical progress and drug use were reviewed in order to assess the outcome.

The main analysis was performed on verbatim consultation transcripts using a modified grounded theory approach, but including ten 'Balint-style' meetings at which the emerging analysis was discussed and different ways of managing specific patients and situations were considered (Balint, 1964; Strauss and Corbin, 1990). Using this inherently flexible approach allowed individual strategies to be developed for each patient, yet the depth of the data gathered allowed causal links to be established in a way that we believe most clinicians will find convincing. Figure 7.1 illustrates diagrammatically how the four main aspects of the study were seen as interdependent.

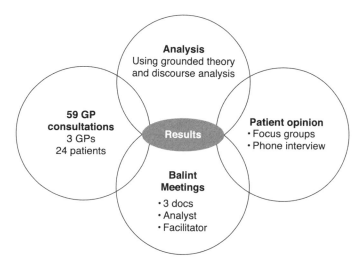

Figure 7.1

The final analysis was a synthesis of the most promising strategies developed, combined with a review of each patient's outcome and view of the process.

In total, 59 consultations were recorded, lasting for between 15 and 40 minutes. As half of the patients showed a substantial improvement in clinical care and almost all perceived their relationship with their doctor to have benefited, it seems that the approach we devised has merit. To explore the limits of the approach, we deliberately included two patients with complex behavior patterns reflecting personality problems, but we failed to constructively engage either of them.

The remainder of this chapter describes our interpretation of the issues related to medication use, the strategies we developed for exploring these issues, and suggestions for managing them. These should not be seen as definitive, but simply as considered suggestions arising after a period of deeply reflective group study and practice.

Figure 7.2 depicts a potentially cyclical journey from the identification of the need for a stronger therapeutic alliance to achieving one. As will by now be clear, this does not necessarily equate with the patient complying with conventional medical practice.

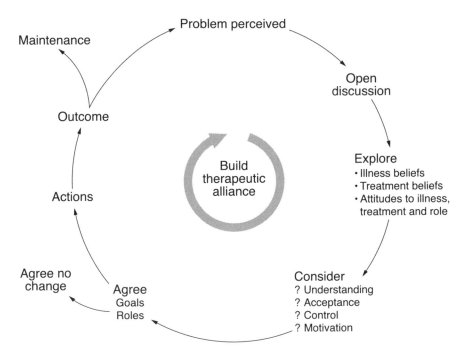

Figure 7.2 The therapeutic alliance model.

It is probably simplest to consider the four key elements in turn – that is, opening discussion, exploring the patient's perspective in detail, considering the potential barriers to constructive medication use, and reaching agreement. Lastly, we should consider how the outcome might be judged in terms of medication decisions or use and the impact on the doctor–patient relationship, because patient-centered care cannot be judged purely by clinical markers.

Opening discussion

Patients can be classified into general groups – those who are eager to 'confess' their medication use, which is helpful and immediately establishes an open relationship, and those who are not. For those who may feel defensive, it is all too easy to initially provoke accounts of *compliance*. Focussing on these can be very problematic. When *non-compliance* is known for sure, these accounts are clearly not true and lead to an uncomfortable and counter-productive discrepancy which traps the patient and hampers the relationship. Having claimed *compliance*, altering their account would reveal the deceit, which is not an easy thing to do in an ostensibly trusting relationship. We tried a confrontational approach with two patients, inviting them to reconcile the prescription record with their account, but found that this merely results in more complex false accounts.

Case example: David

Here are two extracts about David, an undoubtedly *non-compliant* hypertensive patient. First, he claims to *comply*. Inviting him to explain how this could be when the prescribing record indicated so few prescriptions had been issued simply entrenched his position, with exaggerated claims of supplies through a clinical trial. This was only resolved at the end of the fourth and final consultation.

> *Dr Greg: "So can I ask you to run through with me how you actually manage to take ...?"*
> *David: "I take them all in the morning."*
> *Dr Greg: "Right. You just take them all ..."*
> *David: "Eight o'clock every morning."*
> *Dr Greg: "Take them all together."*
> *David: "The wife has them all laid out for me."*
> *Dr Greg: "Right. OK."*
> *David: "So I just take them when I come downstairs."*
> *Dr Greg: "Right. OK. Do you ever forget them?"*
> *David: "No, 'cos the wife ..."*

David's blood pressure control improved immediately, but only after three more consultations was this issue resolved.

> *Dr Greg: "Any idea what was going wrong before?"*
> *David: "Well, remember I stopped my pills when I was feeling great and I stopped them for a while and I think that was the bugbear. And then you put me back on them."*

Although David resumes treatment, the process is suboptimal and frustrating because it is not clear why, and his concerns may not have been adequately dealt with. Failure to achieve open disclosure proved extremely inefficient in this case, as four consultations were required when one or two could have sufficed.

After trying alternative opening strategies, it was concluded that an initial exploration of patients' understanding and beliefs about their condition is most effective. For instance, 'Tell me about when your diagnosis of ... was made' is very informative and effective. Such questions evoke narrative accounts of patients' experiences that reveal associated emotions and often indicate significant barriers to treatment use. Focussing on them, their story and perspective appears to create a climate in which patients feel valued, and enables them to introduce their perspectives gradually. Perhaps this is unsurprising, but it did illustrate to the clinicians involved, all of whom taught patient-centered medicine, the value of starting with the patient's viewpoint. Although perhaps counterintuitive when there was an apparently clear issue around medication use to discuss, a deliberate and extended inquiry into *feelings, ideas, function and expectation (FIFE)* proved to be very efficient use of time.

Examples of helpful probes include the following.

- 'How was your diagnosis made?'
- 'How do you feel about having ...?'
- 'What does this diagnosis mean to you?'
- 'What are the implications for you of having this ...?'

Understanding their perspective naturally produces a patient-centered clinical encounter, as only the patient knows which topics are important to them. Open questions and active listening will be rewarded with efficient exchange of information later on, and the beginnings of an enhanced relationship (Silverman *et al.*, 1998). This obliges the clinician to accept and work with the patient's beliefs and values, but does not prevent them from challenging those beliefs or even, with care, challenging the underlying values.

In Chapter 2 we introduced the story of Susan, who was severely asthmatic. Extracts from her consultations reveal how a more open account can be allowed to emerge using reflective techniques and active listening rather than challenge.

Case example: Susan (continued)

> Susan: *"I mean if I'm told to take them [inhalers] I take them."*
> Dr Rogers: *"OK."*
> Susan: *"I'll admit there are some days I don't think I need them, but I still take them."*
> Dr Rogers: *"What is it that makes you think you don't need them sometimes?"*
> Susan: *"I feel great. I'm not wheezy or anything, but I know that I'm supposed to take them."*

This developed into the following:

> Susan: *"So if I didnae think I needed them, I didnae take them."*
> Dr Rogers: *"So what treatment is it you would miss on these good days?"*
> Susan: *"My inhalers."*
> Dr Rogers: *"Right. How do you know if it's going to be a good day or not?"*
> Susan: *"Depends on how I feel when I get up in the morning."*

The aim of this initial diagnostic phase is to establish how the patient manages their condition and to ascertain whether there is scope for improvement. Do they perceive or construct their illness in a way that is compatible with appropriate care? Or are there substantive differences between clinician and patient understanding that need to be addressed? For instance, a patient who believes that they know when their blood pressure is elevated because they feel tense or have a headache might logically only use treatment at these times. Revealing such discrepancies allows them to be considered.

In addition to exploring the logical or cognitive element of a patient's response to their illness, a patient-centered approach, particularly if it encourages a narrative account, will usually indicate significant underlying emotional responses as well. Substantive anger, or indeed despair, concerning their illness is likely to block medication use as well as other potentially helpful lifestyle changes. This must be identified and explored before discussing the options available.

It is a simple progression from the illness to discussing understanding and beliefs about treatment. Patients may do this spontaneously or it may need to be initiated by the clinician. This is a specific addition to patient-centered diagnostic interviewing, and it should be based on an awareness of the types of roles that patients may play (passively accepting treatment on trust or being a more active decision maker) and the substantive impact that the results of deliberate or incidental medication 'testing' often have. Thus discussing the rationale for medication use usually reveals actual use in a natural and unthreatening fashion. Whether deliberate or accidental experimentation is the source of the rationale also indicates the role that this individual is likely to prefer.

Suitable questions include the following.

- 'Take me back to when you started this ...'
- 'How do you feel about your treatment for ...?'
- 'How do you judge whether it is working?'
- 'Do you have any problems with ...?'

Because it is essential to create an atmosphere in which discussion can be open, and because it is so easy to trap patients into giving reflex accounts that they *comply, it is probably best to avoid direct questions about medication use altogether*. Treatment use will commonly be revealed more honestly while you are exploring how the patient learned what effect the treatment has, without the need for direct questions.

Common problems

We identified four separate problems that could explain medication use within our study group, each of which has been reported previously in the literature on *compliance*. We termed these *understanding, acceptance, control* and *motivation*, and illustrations of each are presented below along with an attempt to describe the type of difficulties they create. Note that all of these patients were known beyond all reasonable doubt to be *non-compliant* (i.e. they were not requesting prescriptions appropriately), so any statements inferring *compliant* treatment use are untrue and indicate that the interaction has not yet reached a satisfactorily open level.

Understanding of illness and treatment

Around one-third of our patients appeared to have an organized but medically inaccurate understanding of their illness or treatment, which led to inappropriate medication management. By this we mean that their perception of the cause of disease, treatment or prognosis for their condition was incorrect. None of these patients were ignorant of the prescription instructions, in terms of dose or frequency – after all, they could always read the label if they were in doubt. Rather their evaluation and subsequent use of treatment was inappropriate because they were judging these by incorrect criteria. They misunderstood the mode of action, potential effects, side-effects, etc., and so made what we saw as poor decisions about treatment use. Personal experience, along with that of others they knew, formed the foundations of these beliefs, which could be helpful or misleading.

This diabetic man does not need to hear more about the long-term effects of diabetes in order to motivate better control. His insights are correct and enhance his motivation:

> *Well, I've had relations who have had diabetes, and they had their legs amputated, they lost their sight. So the fear is there that these things happen.*

By contrast, this man believed that he knew when his blood pressure was elevated, and it is easy to see how symptomatic use of antihypertensive agents would result from this.

> *Doctor: "So do you feel that you can tell when your blood pressure is up?"*
> *Patient: "Yes, I can tell within myself, you know."*
> *Doctor: "Based on what?"*
> *Patient: "My face goes red, you know. And the wife will say to me 'You're blue about here' – you know that's it. ... Blood pressure."*

Misunderstandings are a particular problem in asymptomatic illnesses (such as hypertension) or following an opportunistic diagnosis when emotions may be running high and explanations may be minimal (for example, when surgery is cancelled because of hypertension or diabetes). These are not simple misunderstandings about the regime, or failure to understand instructions, but may concern what the treatment is aimed at, how it works or how it is evaluated. They may also reflect a reluctance to hear information because of an emotive response to the news. Consequently, treatment effects will be incorrectly assessed and appropriate use will be obstructed. This fits entirely with the importance placed on patients' interpretation in the relevant decision-making models that all give the evaluation of treatment a central role (Nerenz and Leventhal, 1983; Meyer *et al.*, 1985; Leventhal *et al.*, 1992; Dowell and Hudson, 1997).

In the following extract, the diagnosis of hypertension is incompletely understood and the persistent use of 'it' and 'this' also suggest that it has not been sufficiently accepted. Therefore intermittent treatment use to please the doctor prior to reviews is not really surprising.

> But like I say, I never gave this a lot of thought. It's never ... it's not something you can see or feel or anything. So I don't have a lot of thoughts about it. I'm not convinced the tablets I'm taking are the right ones I should be taking because it hasn't cured it.

So we have demonstrated that misunderstandings easily arise about both disease and medicines. Therefore when treatment use is a concern it is worth specifically enquiring into beliefs about medication as well as about illness. Unless conflicting beliefs and expectations can be brought into the open and discussed, it is unlikely that much progress will be made.

Case example: Susan (continued)

> Susan's asthma is so severe that she nearly died from a respiratory arrest, which causes both her and her doctors considerable anxiety. Here we see how she improves the way in which she manages her condition. She believes that her asthma is a progressive illness with a distinct endpoint that frightens her.
>
> > *Dr Rogers: "How do you think your condition's going to affect you in the future?"*
> > *Susan: "It's going to put me off my legs. I won't be able to walk."*

The research team conclude that Susan accepts that she has asthma and is well motivated to manage her condition, but that she has become confused in trying to exert some control over her treatment. The task now is to explore and modify her rationale for medication use. At the second meeting, shortly after a further asthma attack, she is more open about her medication use, and this provides an opening for some tailored education about how the inhalers work.

Dr Rogers: "Tell me about the times when you don't take drugs as you're told."
Susan: "Well, say from Saturday. I got up on Saturday morning and took a
Uniphyllin. Now if I feel OK I won't take my inhalers. Maybe come afternoon,
depending on what I'm doing, I'll maybe feel a bit wheezy so I'll go and take one puff
of my inhaler. Then before bed I take two Uniphyllin and I will take my inhaler
again if I think I need it. I take that religiously."
Dr Rogers: "And that's both the inhalers?"
Susan: "Mm."
Dr Rogers: "Do you know how they work and what they do?"

This led to a detailed discussion about how steroid inhalers work. For some reason, possibly the strength of the relationship or perhaps reduced anxiety levels, the information, which must surely have been given before, was absorbed on this occasion. In the extract below this is consolidated by helping to organize an explicit trial of treatment in keeping with the known importance of the medication-testing process.

Dr Rogers: "Have you ever had a spell when you have taken a preventer all the
time, or have you always been a bit iffy about taking them?"
Susan: "Well, as I say, nobody explained to me what they were. So if I didnae think
I needed them I didnae take them."
Dr Rogers: "OK. Then can we see what happens maybe over the next six to eight
weeks with you taking it all the time? We'll see how you are and take it from
there."
Susan: "Yeah. Mm."
Dr Rogers: "Any questions you want to ask me?"
Susan: "No. I think you've clarified that with me, the preventer and the relaxer,
and at least I know what I'm doing now. I know what's for what. What are the
Uniphyllin for?"

Susan's question about Uniphyllin is a positive sign that she is actively engaged in the process, and feels able to reveal her ignorance and resolve her own uncertainties (despite her previous reports that she 'takes Uniphyllin religiously'). At review, after she has been able to reassess her treatment use (a dramatic success) in the light of an improved understanding, she appreciated that this had been a problem. She had had nine emergency admissions with asthma in the previous 3 years, and seven other courses of oral steroids as emergency treatment. In the 4 years following this review she had two admissions and three courses of steroids. As a result she was also able to breed and exercise more horses, which was her main love in life.

In conclusion, the aim of exploring understanding of illness and treatment is to gain insight into how a patient constructs their illness, to help the prescriber to work from and with the patient's views. In terms of the *therapeutic decision model* or the *self-regulatory model*, this recognizes that for *non-compliant* patients, personal experiences of illness and treatment are often the primary influence on their pattern of drug use and their evaluation of treatment (Nerenz and Leventhal, 1983; Meyer *et al.*, 1985; Leventhal *et al.*, 1992; Dowell and Hudson, 1997). However, we found that even patients with pre-existing experience-based beliefs are generally willing to consider further treatment trials when these are proposed in an appropriate atmosphere. In fact, the process of exploring understanding and beliefs using empathic listening techniques appears to allow previously unasked questions to surface, and may be therapeutic in itself. Knowing that your clinician understands your perspective may increase trust and facilitate repeated and more supervised therapeutic experimentation in collaboration between patient and clinician. This process facilitates a sense of partnership.

Acceptance of illness and treatment

The second problem that we identified was acceptance. One way of coping with a threat is to attempt to ignore it or play it down, and such behavior is particularly notable in patients with devastating diagnoses, when this coping mechanism may be termed denial. Although avoidance behaviors such as this may help an individual to cope in the short term, they do not help constructive adjustments to be made to long-term illness. This psychological mechanism is also employed in less threatening medical situations, and can influence treatment use and other behaviors. Adjusting to any illness requires some degree of acceptance, and although conditions such as hypertension, diabetes and even asthma may not be obvious or seen as serious, they may still challenge an individual's view of him- or herself. Acceptance is not the same as letting the illness rule life, but rather it is an adjustment that allows accommodation so that the rest of life can continue. Acknowledging a condition that requires lifelong medication or behavior change is an emotional event that patient-centered prescribing should recognize. So avoiding medicines might be a sign of failure or ineffective adjustment to illness. However, a patient may fully acknowledge their illness without necessarily agreeing to take a specific treatment, and they are entitled to have their views or concerns respected without being labelled as 'in denial.' The act of taking medication can be quite symbolic and may have a potent metaphorical role (Montagne, 1988). There are also many studies which have reported that people dislike and distrust modern medicines, and the phrase 'I don't take medicines unless I have to' must be internationally recognisable (Horne, 1997; Horne and Weinman, 1999). The problem is the 'have to.' How can clinicians know or recognize when an illness has been sufficiently accepted, and how can we help those who are struggling to accept the need for a treatment that could benefit them?

Just as directly enquiring about medication use is often ineffective, so is a direct enquiry about denial/acceptance. Not only might the patient resent being asked such a potentially threatening question, but also they may not have considered or indeed be able to reflect on this adequately themselves. It is unlikely that a useful reply will be obtained.

Again it seems that the basic patient-centered technique of eliciting views and beliefs about the condition and – we would again add – about treatment, proves very effective. The clinician merely has to be tuned to the appropriate clues. Although patients may explicitly express anger or denial, the tone and language that they use to describe their situation is often more informative in this regard than the content. Another indicator is the way in which they have adapted functionally. Adaptation to illness may be reflected in physical, psychological or social adjustment, which might, respectively, be represented by changes in activities, being able to calmly discuss their condition or being open about it with others (such as friends or employers). Conversely, signs of strong emotions, resistance to making necessary adjustments (possibly including treatment use) or trying to socially conceal the illness might all raise suspicions that this issue is blocking a constructive response. This requires some judgement, as clearly not everyone will or should want to discuss their medical condition widely.

We found inviting a narrative account to be the most helpful approach, enhanced by using open questions about feelings to expand accounts. So the same starts could glean useful information about both understanding and acceptance of illness and treatment. Typical phrases include the following.

- 'Take me back to when you first found you had ...'
- 'What happened when this treatment was first suggested?'

Helpful probes include the following.

- 'So how do you feel about that?'
- 'What impact did that have on you?'

Discussing the moment of the initial diagnosis is the most revealing time for assessing how far someone has come to terms with their situation. Effective acceptance may be represented by constructive adjustments, such as medication use becoming comfortably habitual, as well as an absence of resentment or bitterness reflected in the tone and language used. Another linguistic sign of acceptance is when medication or illnesses are described using a personal pronoun, such as 'my', implying a sense of ownership, as opposed to the indefinite article, 'it', implying distance. Compare the following extracts:

> ... since I had **the illness**, you know. Never bothered about tablets. **It** doesn't worry me at all.

> **My** diabetes doesn't affect me all that much.

Although acceptance might by definition be seen as a psychological process, the physical and social markers of acceptance provide useful indicators. Physically adapting life in a sensible way that accommodates the restrictions enforced by illness suggests a constructive psychological response. Again this is particularly convincing if the language used makes this adaptation seem willing, as illustrated by the following quote.

> It doesn't restrict my day-to-day living. Over the years I have limited the type of sports I do. Because I've had it for so long. I don't know whether I really see it as an illness. It's part of my life.

This patient has accepted asthma as part of her way of life, and is apparently at ease with the situation. The adaptations do not necessarily have to be ideal from the medical perspective, but the fact that they are willingly made suggests that the individual has come to terms with their situation – it has become 'part of life.'

By contrast, another asthmatic patient is so reluctant to accept her inhalers that she makes unnecessary lifestyle changes and trades symptoms against medication use as she perceives the relative threats of each very differently from her doctor. The way in which she apparently willingly adapts life to her asthma rather than using inhalers suggests that the main issue is with accepting the medication rather than the condition. It transpires that this is due to fear of side-effects.

> That would be asking for trouble. I wouldn't aggravate the problem. I wouldn't encourage myself to have to take my inhaler. I have all day to do things, taking the longer walk for the exercise and going up the lesser hill, I wouldn't need to take my inhaler. I haven't done anything strenuous and I've still got to where I need to, but I've not hurt myself in doing it.

Another asthmatic patient who fights against treatment and clinicians provides our most extreme example of denial, which he illustrates in terms of both psychological and social indicators. He constantly tries to work harder to overcome his illness and conceal his diagnosis from others. His reluctance to accept his illness is also reflected in his preference for medication in tablet form because he is embarrassed about his inhaler, indicating his lack of social adjustment.

> Probably, because of my asthma, I do more work than somebody else. Because you're trying to prove that it doesn't hold you back. It makes you understand why people will lie sometimes about their health. I certainly would never put it on a form.

> I used to carry these inhalers about with me you know and they were rattling. These blinking inhalers and it's embarrassing. Even though I've had asthma all my life it's still a bit embarrassing taking inhalers. That's why I wanted to go on to something that people don't see [treatment in tablet form].

Contrast this with a patient who demonstrates how an accepted treatment, in this case salbutamol, might be managed.

> There's one [inhaler] in my handbag, one in my pocket and there's one in the medicine drawer.

In conclusion, accepting illness is difficult at times, and reluctance to take treatment can reflect this, as can other physical and social indicators. In addition, an illness may be accepted but the suggested treatment may not. Although clinicians may feel uncomfortable initiating discussion on sensitive topics like this, an exploration of the patient's experience to date will often provide sufficient information without the need for direct questions. Denial of illness may sometimes be a healthy and adaptive response, and forcing patients to overcome such barriers may counter patient-centered principles and could be counterproductive. However, if denial blocks therapeutic interventions it can lead to problems, and therefore it becomes the clinician's responsibility to help where they can. Clearly, different approaches are likely to be required, so identifying as accurately as possibly where the problem lies is important. Looking at X-rays, investigation results, peak flow charts or home blood pressure recordings might help to establish the disease, about which the patient has no choice. However, this may have little impact on getting a treatment accepted if the problem stems from concerns about side-effects or addiction. Making sure that the patient is aware of the alternatives in an environment where they are free to exert their choice would seem to be the least that is compatible with good care. How you can attempt to do this is described in more detail later in this chapter under 'Vignettes of negotiation.'

Control over management

Some patients want active control over their management, whereas others seem content to play a passive role. In the literature on shared decision making this is termed 'role preference.' However, the level of control that a patient wants can be very difficult to ascertain. Some will indicate a clear desire to be involved by taking the initiative, asking questions and informing themselves from the outset. Indeed, these assertive patients may be the only ones who currently really participate in the decision-making process. Eliciting a patient's role preference is heavily dependent on the tone of the interaction. As has already been discussed, the current behavioral norms in medical encounters tend to disempower patients, and this situation needs to be deliberately overcome as far as possible to enable patients to contribute. A token enquiry in the midst of an interview that is clearly being led by the clinician is unlikely to encourage the patient to assert him- or herself and assume a substantive role. Again the patient-centered approach will assist this process, but it may also help to use visual scales so that the patient can indicate their preference without necessarily verbalising it. Two such scales are shown in Figures 7.3 and 7.4.

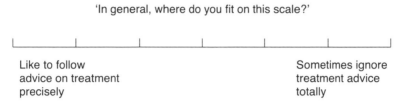

Figure 7.3

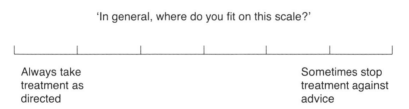

Figure 7.4

Even using such scales, the customary reluctance to admit *non-compliance* or demand control needs to be accounted for. Only those who indicate the far left, *compliant* ends of the scales are likely to be passive by choice. Patients who actively adapt advice tend to indicate a central position, while those who wish to make a clear statement or be provocative may indicate the far right ends of the scales.

> Doctor: *"If we look at this, medication use in general, where do you fit on this scale?"*
> Patient: *"Somewhere in the middle, I think. Probably bang in the middle because it depends what it is. It depends how I feel about it I suppose, or how it makes me feel."*

This reply reflects an active patient but not a confrontational one, and provides an opening for further clarification, perhaps regarding a specific treatment, or exploring the feeling in more detail. Patients are usually cautious about admitting that they ignore advice, but the above scales can provide an easy way of generating discussion. Medication use can also be indicative of the control that they wish to assume, and this can complicate the clinical relationship if it is not matched by the clinician. This appeared to be a problem for about one-third of our study patients. In general this is because an active patient's desire for control exceeds what their doctor offers. These conflicts reflect an immature clinical relationship, where manipulative behaviors are likely to be employed before collaborative ones. Intentional *non-compliance* is one very powerful way in which a patient can exert their control over that of the clinician, so it is prudent to at least consider this dimension of the relationship when it is encountered.

> Patient: *"Sometimes, when I take the medicine, say you've upped it to 50 mg. Now when I take them. I took it for six days ... 50 and then I thought, well, I'm a bit tired, so the next day I halved it. That's experience."*

Some patients' experimentation and subsequent *non-compliance* with their medication results in them being considered 'difficult.' It is perhaps more constructive to see them as simply indicating a desire to be active participants in their care.

Apart from *non-compliance*, a questioning attitude also implies that a patient is or wants to be active. An inquisitive individual is more likely to become well informed and make sensible decisions about their healthcare as a result, so this should be encouraged. All of the following extracts are positive signs that these different patients are becoming engaged in their healthcare when they had not been previously:

> "I'd like to know more if possible."

> "What causes ... what is causing the high blood pressure then?"

> "The tablets I'm on ... is it putting my pressure down?"

By helping patients to manage their treatments constructively, more mature therapeutic relationships can be established and tensions can be resolved. However, at the other end of the spectrum the patient's desire for control may actually fall as the relationship develops and they prefer a more directive style. These 'passive' patients are worth special consideration. The following consultation extracts are typical of early accounts of compliance:

> "Now I just go along with what you've prescribed."

> "If it's going to help me then fair and well."

These patients imply that they are taking their medication accurately, yet they are known not to be doing so. By definition, such *non-compliance* can be interpreted as not accepting treatment passively, and suggests a desire to exert control. Possibly handing over control to the doctor is a coping mechanism that avoids the need to fully acknowledge their situation. However, this has to be questioned, as these individuals are neither using treatment effectively nor willing to discuss it openly. It is not a helpful response, and it implies that the clinician might have postponed or avoided the questions about medication use that tend to prompt these reflex accounts of *compliance*.

Clearly there are patients who wish the clinician to make all of the decisions. This might apply to any individual at times of crisis when they feel particularly vulnerable and overwhelmed, but some patients also appear to genuinely want to play a passive role. However, identifying these individuals correctly may be complicated because of their past interactions with the medical profession. There are two main possibilities. First, the clinician may have failed to adequately convey their desire for a collaborative relationship, and the patient remains trapped in a deferential position, unable to voice their opinions or take control as they wish. This implies insufficient skill on the practitioner's part, or a failure to appreciate the power imbalance as perceived by the patient – a dangerous trap, but easy to fall into. Secondly, the desire to remain passive may indicate that the patient feels overwhelmed by their current situation, even when this is a chronic illness without immediate threat to life.

Case example: Bill

In the following extract, Bill, a diabetic, confirms that this he wants to remain passive in three ways:

> Dr Jack: *"Now there seem to be three real kind of routes through which people go. There are some people who say 'Right, I'm not taking any tablets. I don't want to do that.' Which doesn't sound like you?"*
>
> Bill: *"No, I'll take any tablet."*
>
> Dr Jack: *"And there are others who say 'Right doc, whatever you say, that's fine.' But the majority seem to go through a process of trying their drugs out, seeing if they suit them, seeing if they think they work well for them and then deciding in the end how they are going to use them for themselves. Now I know you're not in this category, but which of these do you feel you might be in?"*
>
> Bill: *"This one"* [indicating passive compliance on scale].
>
> Dr Jack: *"You feel that you're fairly passive about the way that you ...?"*
>
> Bill: *"Yes, aha."*
>
> Dr Jack: *"And do you feel happy about doing it that way?"*
>
> Bill: *"Yes, anytime, I'm happy as far as my health goes."*
>
> Dr Jack: *"Right. You'd prefer to just hand it over and let the doc ...?"*
>
> Bill: *"Hand over and let the doctor deal with it. Well, we're under your care so ..."*
>
> Dr Jack: *"Sure?"*
>
> Bill: *"It's what I look for."*
>
> Dr Jack: *"Is that the way you would sort of address other things in your life? If you were going to get an insurance premium or something would you just take the advice and say 'Right, OK. I've found some advice. If that's what you say I'll do it'?"*
>
> Bill: *"Yeah."*
>
> Dr Jack: *"You're happy with that sort of approach?"*
>
> Bill: *"Mm, yes."*
>
> Dr Jack: *"OK."*

In conclusion, patients vary in the level of control that they want or appear to take over their situation. In some cases this is obvious – for example, a patient demanding a specific treatment. However, others wish to present themselves as passive, *compliant* treatment users when this is clearly not the case. We must conclude that this is difficult territory for some patients to discuss openly, even within deliberately empathic and extended consultations. Using tools such as visual scales may help, but the risk of falsely accepting that a patient prefers a passive role is substantial unless great care is taken to establish a supportive atmosphere and assess their preferences carefully. This reflects the global assumption underlying the entire *compliance* paradigm – that patients want to do what the doctor advises but just need help to understand and follow the instructions!

Motivation

There are patients who sincerely wish to control their illnesses better and are happy with the guidance they have received, but cannot manage to achieve that control. This was described in Chapter 3 according to the *theory of planned behavior* when 'intention to act' fails to be converted into 'action.' It can then be very tempting to blame patients for simply not trying hard enough, but in our study only two of the 22 patients appeared to be in this situation. These two diabetic men were quite open about their inability to control their diet tightly, and reported inconsistent medication use because they gave up, feeling hopeless about their poor management. Interestingly, the clinicians whom they met who emphasized this poor control appeared to only exaggerate their failings and demotivate them further. This itself deterred them from attending for review and reinforced their view that they might as well not try. Both of these patients requested specific, directive instructions to overcome their motivational difficulties, and seemed to feel reluctant to accept greater personal responsibility for their health.

Case example: Bill (continued)

> Bill: "It [treatment] works for a few weeks and then it ..."
> Dr Jack: "Yeah, OK. So it's not that you've got a big problem with the ..."
> Bill: "... advice ... it's just carrying it out."

Concluding that someone's primary problem is an inability to adhere to an understood and accepted treatment plan should really be seen as a diagnosis of last resort. Before this conclusion can be reached, it is necessary to ensure that understanding, acceptance and control are not the problem. During this process it should be apparent that the clinical goals are valued and accepted (i.e. they are seen as 'important'; Rollnick *et al.*, 1999). However, 'confidence' in their ability to achieve the necessary progress is likely to be very low. These can also usefully be assessed on visual scales.

For these patients, additional information about the risks is not helpful, nor is being obliged to make their own decisions about treatment. Both may be overwhelming and counterproductive. Their low confidence may make it impossible for them to take control, and leaves them feeling unable to achieve the targets that they accept are important. They require specific help with achieving lifestyle changes in a way that enhances confidence.

Summary of assessment of your patient

The message that this section has sought to convey has two primary components. First, there are a variety of reasons why patients get into difficulties as a result of ineffective treatment use. These require different responses to help them to progress, and blaming patients, or issuing threats about dire consequences, tends to be counterproductive. Secondly, falling back on a patient-centered approach by trying to sensitively under-
ation from their perspective will at least be informative, and is sometimes own right. To achieve this requires a genuinely safe atmosphere where ble to discuss *non-compliance* and to consider the implications that taking sibility might have for them. This requires an investment in relationship nts whose treatment use is not optimal have to be encouraged to assume

responsibility for their treatment, which may mean choosing not to follow established best practice, or perhaps electing not to take treatment at all. Depending on the nature of the condition, this may require a substantial shift in attitude on the part of the clinician. As we progress into the therapeutic component or intervention process, it is important to revisit the underlying ethos on which this approach is founded, because clinicians who are unwilling to let patients manage their own care (within some limits) (*see* Chapter 6) risk falling into a form of manipulation, with limited hope of success and a risk of further damaging a weak therapeutic relationship.

The Royal Pharmaceutical Society of Great Britain working party report has challenged professionals to adapt to the changing nature of the doctor–patient relationship (Blenkinsopp *et al.*, 1997). It introduced the term concordance, which it defined as follows:

> The clinical encounter is concerned with two sets of contrasted but equally cogent health beliefs – that of the patient and that of the prescriber. The task of the patient is to convey his or her health beliefs to the prescriber, and that of the prescriber, to enable this to happen. The task of the prescriber is to convey his or her (professionally informed) health beliefs to the patient and of the patient to entertain these. The intention is to assist the patient to make as informed a choice as possible about the diagnosis and treatment, about benefit and risk, and to take full part in a therapeutic alliance. **Although reciprocal, this is an alliance in which the most important determinations are agreed to be those that are made by the patient.**

This landmark shift in the approach to prescribing practice has two small inconsistencies in its definition that seem to make it difficult for some to accept this concept. First, it may be problematic for some to consider the beliefs of the prescriber and the patient as being '*equally cogent.*' The *Oxford English Dictionary* defines cogent as 'convincing' or 'compelling', but most people would recognize that the increasing body of scientific knowledge underpinning western medicine is more convincing than any one individual's beliefs. The patient's beliefs may be of equal *importance* because of their ability to affect treatment use, but should not necessarily be accepted as equally *cogent*, as this may ostracize many healthcare professionals and ignore the benefits of medical advances. Secondly, patients are rarely in a position to make an informed choice about their diagnosis, although the importance of their desire to do so is not questioned.

In response to these observations, a more useful working definition may be as follows:

> The professional explores the patient's beliefs about their illness and treatment before ensuring that they appreciate any necessary additional details, risks or options. The professional highlights discrepancies in the patient's situation and helps them to choose a response. Treatment goals are established for both parties before management is agreed. Concordance has not been achieved if significant disparity exists between the two parties' view of the problem, treatment goals or solution. **Where this occurs, the patient's view takes priority unless they are not competent to do so.** Both definitions are based upon and explicitly emphasize the fundamental belief that this process is focussed on helping patients to make informed choices, not getting them to follow professional advice. This requires the clinician to be prepared to let go. They must be willing to let the patient make what they might consider to be the 'wrong' decision. All experienced healthcare professionals will have encountered situations where patients go

against advice, but this is different. Here the clinician is helping or sharing in the decision-making process, not simply arguing their corner. This does not mean that they hold no view about the best course of action, but that they recognize the patient's authority to decide for him- or herself. Note that a patient cannot be 'non-concordant', as this describes the relationship. Discord may remain, but this is a shared responsibility. However, they may agree a course of action and then fail to act accordingly. They may fail to 'comply' with or 'adhere' to an agreed plan just as much as to a dictated one. Using a separate term such as 'discrepant' use might help to avoid confusion here. Chapter 8 discusses how clinicians may wish to safeguard themselves against accusations of sanctioning or encouraging decisions that go against current best practice.

Part 2: Vignettes of negotiation

The next part of this chapter discusses how the consultation process may evolve following the exploratory process outlined above, and offers examples from some pragmatic attempts to help patients to develop a constructive approach to managing their illness. Potential ways are presented in which problems identified during the diagnostic process described in Chapter 5 can be addressed. The process of seeking and establishing a shared clinical decision will be described, and the difficult balance between information provision and patient manipulation will be discussed. The process of establishing the patient's preferred role during subsequent consultations and patient-centered goals for treatment use are also included here.

Earlier in this chapter, shared decision making was described on the assumption that there is a fairly clean slate – that patients' opinions and actions are not substantively informed or governed by previous experience, emotions or behavior patterns. However, such complications are the norm when addressing existing patterns of ineffective medication use. Therefore even greater care is required when approaching these situations.

Four separate issues have been suggested as being worth exploring when patients report or are found to be having difficulty using treatments in a medically appropriate way:

- the patient's beliefs about the illness and treatment
- their acceptance of illness and treatment
- their preference for control of their care
- their motivation or ability to achieve their desired health-related behaviors.

Exploring these issues is often challenging, as they involve sensitive areas of patients' beliefs that sometimes conflict with the medical model, and which clinicians may feel are unfamiliar ground or even irrational or irritating behavior. However, identifying and exploring such feelings is an essential component of practicing patient-centered medicine as it is defined within this book series. It is not sufficient to ignore the suboptimal care that is being delivered, or to simply burden the patient with 'the facts' and leave them to resolve the conflict in a potentially adversarial context. The minutiae of such complex interpersonal interactions are extremely difficult to dissect and research in a meaningful way using quantitative approaches. Consequently, there is little of what some would see as firm evidence about the detail of how these issues should be explored

or addressed. However, qualitative approaches are offering incr'
which components of interactions have what effects. Using these m
possible to suggest techniques that clinicians may wish to use and with
develop their skills. As their successful application is so dependent upon the cu
unlikely that substantive trials could ever be completed on the individual techni
described. However, sufficient evidence of effect can be rapidly apparent when successful behavior change is achieved with a few individuals whose longstanding care has
been suboptimal. Rescuing someone who is trapped in an unhelpful pattern of medication use is an extremely rewarding process. Hopefully this book has convinced you
that experimenting with these techniques is a risk worth taking to enhance your own
repertoire of skills.

Misunderstanding

Misunderstandings commonly arise during communication with patients, and two of
the basic manoeuvres suggested when giving information are to check the recipient's
starting point, and to ask for the information to be summarized to demonstrate that
it was accurately received (Silverman *et al.*, 1998; Britten *et al.*, 2000). The process
of discussing treatment acts to review the success with which information has been
assimilated. It also helps to set the level at which further information should be
proffered, without necessarily formally enquiring about preferences for information
provision. This is likely to be especially useful if the rationale for actions is probed, rather
than simply checking that the patient knows what the instructions were. In the
following section we shall dissect out contrasting types of knowledge and suggest
that simple information, however well presented, is not always sufficient to change
behavior. An alternative is to identify what the misunderstanding is based on and to
consider changes or experiments that patients could implement on a trial basis which
are likely to rectify this and inform more constructive treatment use.

Beate *et al.* (1997) describe two types of knowledge – *operational* and *functional*.
Operational knowledge is primarily based on experience and is more likely to influence
action – somewhat akin to so-called 'deep' learning. Functional knowledge is more
superficial – the ability to recall information or instructions. In order to access a
patient's operational knowledge, it helps to ask what they think, feel and do, rather than
what they recall or know.

For instance, compare the following examples:

> Doctor: *"You mentioned that you increased your steroid inhaler when you get
> tight. How do you use it?"*
> Patient: *"Well, I increase it to four times a day as the nurse suggested."*
> Doctor: *"Good. That is a very sensible way to respond ..."*
>
> Doctor: *"You mentioned that you increased your steroid inhaler when you get
> tight. Can you explain how you decide what to do?"*
> Patient: *"Well, when I'm really bad the salbutamol one doesn't seem to work so
> well, and eventually I need to increase the steroids. Sometimes it gets quite
> frightening and I should probably do it sooner."*
> Doctor: *"Why do you say that?"*
> Patient: *"Well, I don't like taking the steroids so I wait until I am really bad. I'd
> prefer to do without them altogether."*
> Doctor: *"Could you tell me more about why that is?"*

In the second example, useful information is revealed that indicates the patient's stance towards the steroids rather than their recall of instructions. By exploring this dislike it may be possible to identify and discuss the specific causes so that both clinician and patient can re-evaluate the medication use with these insights. In effect this is simply employing open questions to help to elucidate the thinking underlying the patient's actions. This usually reveals elements of knowledge or beliefs about their condition and treatment as well as more details about how they manage them. Although occasionally there is a communication failure or misunderstanding that can be simply corrected, more commonly there is a misinterpretation of risk, symptoms or expected benefits for a recognisable reason. For instance, patients who are diagnosed with hypertension who do not attend for review after their first trial of treatment rarely do so because of the stated simple misunderstanding 'I thought it was just a course, doctor.' There are more complex beliefs or anxieties behind such innocent explanations.

A number of techniques have been found to be useful when explaining clinical information, arguably the single most important of which is finding out where the recipient is starting from (Silverman *et al.*, 1998). When patients seem to be using treatments in a suboptimal way due to such misinterpretations, any effective response should be based upon the cause of this, not simply a reiteration of the instructions, however carefully delivered. Of course people value their own experiences more strongly than advice from others, and beliefs based upon experience may well require a contrasting experience before they can be recast. Therefore it can be helpful to invite and guide a further trial of treatment in the hope of achieving a more favourable outcome, rather than to imply that the patient has made a mistake and should now fall into line with conventional medical wisdom. Although this technique is particularly helpful when symptom control can be assessed, or even some form of monitoring employed, it can still be used to assess side-effects for almost all medicines.

Case example: Jackie

When Jackie, an asthmatic woman, sought a repeat prescription, it was noticed that she used regular salbutamol (an immediate bronchodilator) but took very little beclomethasone (a steroid preventive inhaler). As she did not attend regularly, she was invited for a review. Jackie had a good understanding of her asthma and accepted it fully – for instance, calling her illness 'mine' ('*my asthma went through a bad time*') and keeping medication in many different places. Indeed her life had been physically redefined by it. She avoided strenuous activity, extending her children's walk to school to use a flat route, and using regular swimming to control her symptoms. She resisted treatment with steroids for fear of '*being dependent on it*', and also due to her previous experience of weight gain with steroids. Jackie wished to control her medication fully. She was given information about the potential value of a more prolonged trial and reassured about the risks of dependency and weight gain with inhaled products, but her resistance to them was not openly confronted. Instead the therapeutic relationship created enough trust for her to be asked to experiment again. She proceeded, with encouragement, to re-engage and test a low dose of inhaled steroids (her preference), and concluded that they were effective and tolerable for her. She then experimented further and now uses conventional doses, but for winter periods only. Her symptom control has improved substantively, and she has maintained control over her steroid use. Her previous problems with weight gain did not recur.

Acceptance

Accepting illness appears to be a difficulty for some individuals, and reluctance to take treatment can reflect this. Accepting an illness or disability of any type requires some adjustment of self-image, and if substantial this may be unpleasant and therefore avoided (Markus and Wurf, 1997). As medicines to some extent symbolize illness, taking less treatment can symbolize less illness, which consequently lessens the challenge to one's self-image. This reflects a mix of cognitive and emotional responses, which is an important aspect of Leventhal's *self-regulatory model* (*see* Chapter 4). This may provide some explanation for life-threatening *non-compliance* (e.g. immunosuppressants not being taken after transplant surgery), as managing without medicines may symbolize a return to normality (Laederach-Hofmann and Bunzel, 2000). Addressing such psychological conflict requires more than mere information (Rollnick *et al.,* 1993). In this section we shall explore the difficulties inherent in creating acceptance. We acknowledge that this is often challenging and emotive, and we suggest that more can be gained by explicitly handing over responsibility for decisions or assessing readiness to change, rather than blaming the patient or implying that they are not being sensible.

   The point at which a patient considers changing their stance can be an awkward one. In our research group we termed this the 'discomfort zone', which largely reflected our own awareness that the interaction had reached a critical and slightly unstable point. This phenomenon of 'reactance arousal' is recognized within psychodynamic therapy and 'is a cornerstone of both the theory and the therapy' (Brehm, 1981). Balint also reported finding that a crisis in the clinical relationship was sometimes instrumental in progress being made (Balint, 1964). So it can be predicted that clinicians will have to manage this type of response or moment. The *readiness to change model* suggests that a nudge in a constructive direction can be effective if it is made at a time when the patient is receptive, but doing so obviously requires care, because of the harm it may cause to the relationship (Prochaska and DiClemente, 1983). There is obviously a fine line between directive advice and unwelcome instruction (Stott and Pill, 1990). For instance, routine advice to stop smoking in primary care was seen as inappropriate and potentially damaging, yet tailored advice from a doctor is probably the most effective single prompt known (Butler *et al.,* 1998). The knack may be in judging when a patient is open to the suggestion of change and whether the 'therapeutic relationship' is sufficiently strong to keep them on side with the clinician. Such psychotherapeutic interactions are not described in any detail within the main texts on primary care consultations, but key skills are considered to be avoiding resistance while helping the individual to become aware of discrepancies or conflicts between their behaviors and their underlying value systems, beliefs and identity. It is achieved in the context of a strong therapeutic relationship by directed reflective listening. Interested readers are referred to Miller and Rollnick (1991) or McDermott and Jago (2001).

Case example: Joan

   Joan's attitude towards her treatment for high blood pressure is explored, indicating what we termed the 'discomfort zone', where crucial emotions were aired and progress was often made. Her apparent irritation probably accounts for her intolerance of all the medicines previously tried.

Dr Brown: "So what are we going to do?"

Joan: "I'm doing fine as I am, aren't I? I've had no dire effects or ... can I say I think the treatment of hypertension and blood pressure is fashionable just now. It's easy for doctors."

Dr Brown: "It's easy for doctors ..."

Joan: "Easy for doctors ... 'Take a pill and come back.' '

Dr Brown: "Right. Tell me about that."

Joan: "Well, that is how I feel. It's easy for patients to come. You don't do anything, nothing unpleasant happens, just take the pill and come back again. Everybody's happy."

Dr Brown: "But you're not happy."

Joan: "I'm not happy taking pills if I don't need them."

Dr Brown: "Right. You sound a bit annoyed about it."

Joan: "No, I'm not annoyed. But I think you've to have it in perspective. I could come every month and say 'Oh, I'm feeling a bit low' and you would be more worried and I would be more worried because I have to come. It requires ... what can I say ... me to think now 'Am I ill enough to go and see Doctor ... or can I just think what I'm about?' And I also consider that I eat too much. I don't think I'm terribly overweight, but I think if I ate less my whole system wouldn't have to work as hard."

Dr Brown: "We talked about how the risks of having a stroke and having problems with your heart and kidney are higher than normal if you have a raised blood pressure. But if you'd rather have these risks ... you've talked before of how you didn't feel it was going to happen to you. "

Joan: "Well, I don't ... I have no symptoms at all. I twigged this blood pressure complaint myself, so what else ... how else ... I don't have headaches. What else would I know about?"

Dr Brown: "They often don't give you symptoms. It's just a question that over time your blood pressure can cause problems with your eyes and with your kidneys."

Joan: "But I would know ..."

Dr Brown: "You would know ... well, you might know, but it's worth having things like blood checked from time to time and to have your urine checked from time to time and your blood pressure."

Joan: "Which I have done this summer."

Dr Brown: "So I think it's maybe worth checking that every six months or every year just to keep an eye on it. To check that those complications aren't arising."

Joan: "Yes, yes."

Dr Brown: "Does that seem a reasonable compromise? Because I think we've been through lots of different combinations of treatment ..."

Joan: "Now would you say that I am medium, poor or good with the blood pressure? My blood pressure – is it in the poor range requiring more treatment or if it's good, I can trot along like this?"

Dr Brown: "I would prefer if you had more treatment."

Joan: "Ah, but you're the doctor."

This woman had tried many medicines for her hypertension, but eventually elected to primarily use diet and exercise to maintain her health and to accept the risks from her condition. She accepted the value of monitoring, and the relationship with her practitioner improved. Some months later a friend had a stroke, which made her feel more vulnerable, and she returned willing to resume treatment. Her doctor thought that she probably would not have done so if the clinical relationship had not been improved.

In this context 'discomfort' is not necessarily produced by confrontation, but can result from the discrepancy between the patient's treatment goals and related behaviors being revealed. The technique of 'developing discrepancy' is an important component of motivational interviewing – one of the best known approaches for achieving health behavior change (Miller and Rollnick, 1991).

A lack of acceptance is often termed denial, but patients rarely deny the possibility that they have a particular condition altogether. Rather, they fail to be fully convinced that they have it or to recognize the implications that it may have. It is then not logical to use treatment, as this does not make sense for a condition they do not have or which they feel that they are managing satisfactorily already (Dowell and Hudson, 1997). As mentioned above, this should be considered when patients use language that dissociates them from the condition (e.g. 'This asthma thing'). When suspected, they will often be pleased to explain why they do not believe they have the condition, which can then lead on to further discussion. Of course some diagnoses are wrong, and at times it will be important to arrange further investigations to check this. On other occasions it can help to use investigations or trials of treatment in a collaborative way to help to convince the patient, even if the clinician has no doubts. This is relatively simple with symptomatic conditions, but is also possible with conditions such as hypertension or diabetes that can be monitored, provided that the patient values the clinical outcome. When necessary, the same markers can also be used to convince patients of the need for treatment using explicit tests on and off therapy. Preventive treatments that cannot be monitored, such as prophylactic aspirin, present a greater challenge. However, simply identifying the issue and allowing the patient to find their own way to overcome the problem can be surprisingly effective. It seems enough for some patients to express their beliefs for their level of acceptance to improve, and it may help to simply have their concerns about side-effects or other issues voiced and acknowledged.

When there is an apparent impasse it can be tempting to feel that the patient is to blame for not recognising the facts as interpreted by the clinician. However, it has been suggested that denial can be intensified by implying that a patient is not cooperating with the clinician (Ness, 1994). Confrontation is a high-risk strategy which is certainly likely to strain the clinical relationship. An alternative, more productive approach whenever a stalemate develops is to review the patient's therapeutic goals and to reconsider how these can best be achieved. Common ground can usually be established in this way and the negative effects of direct confrontation avoided. The clinician's goals then take second place but are rarely excluded altogether.

Case example: Mrs Tait

Mrs Tait, an elderly woman who had been receiving treatment for hypertension for many years, was noted to have collected far too few prescriptions over the last few years. At review it became apparent that she did not really believe that she had high blood pressure. She felt that she knew when she was 'tensed up', and she used her treatment for a few days when this was the case. Although she attended the surgery and had a record of persistently high readings, she did not want additional treatment. It became apparent that she did not believe the readings were a true reflection of her usual blood pressure, although the consistency of the readings had convinced her doctor of her diagnosis. To resolve this discrepancy, Mrs Tait was loaned a home blood pressure monitor and took a series of her own readings. Through this she came to recognize that she could not accurately sense her blood pressure and that it was genuinely elevated. Consequently, she decided to use her treatment regularly.

Case example: Tom

Another patient, Tom, was reluctant to accept that he had hypertension and in particular hypercholesterolemia (which had been diagnosed some years earlier and medication commenced), perhaps due to their asymptomatic nature. At the first consultation Tom stated:

> Well, I never knew I had high cholesterol. It didnae effect me at all as far as I was aware. I'm quite happy because it doesn't seem to affect me. The cholesterol ... so I'm quite happy, I am with that like.

In the second consultation he began to ask questions and became more engaged:

> Dr Henry: "All right. The other thing was your cholesterol."
> Tom: "Aye. It was up. I take it that's because of what I eat?" ....
> Tom: "The tablets I take for blood pressure, does that also go for cholesterol as well. Does it no help?" ...
> Tom: "The exercise is going to help though, right?"
> Dr Henry: "Perhaps what we should do with your cholesterol is give you some advice about the diet and then check your cholesterol again in three months' time."

The doctor had succeeded in challenging this patient's denial or avoidance of the cholesterol problem simply by making him aware of his concern. By the second consultation, the patient's attitude had changed and he was willing to act. He had already expressed and demonstrated a dislike of tablets, but was willing to exercise and diet. The doctor emphasized the need for monitoring to reinforce the presence of the condition as a prelude to possibly suggesting drug therapy again in the future.

Control

This section highlights the difficulty of meaningfully judging such a fluid and vague concept as control or 'role preference', especially within a clinical encounter. The value of offering control is demonstrated through case examples, even though explicit requests for greater control are rare. Perhaps it should always be offered to those who demonstrate ineffective medication use.

There is a wealth of psychological literature examining the extent to which individuals seek to control their lives, including their health. This has been assimilated into the models of decision making, usually under the term 'role preference.' After all, it would not be very patient-centered to insist that someone made their own decision when they wished the clinician to do so for them. Thus models of shared decision making include a stage of eliciting the patient's preferred role in the decision-making process – itself an inexact process, as many people do not have a clear view of the role that they wish to play, and it may vary as the relationship deepens or the implications of the decision become apparent. There is limited evidence that people who are happy with their involvement in the decision-making process are more likely to subsequently act on their decision (O'Connor *et al.*, 2003a).

Stewart and others have advocated a relationship based on 'mutuality' that necessitates the active involvement of both parties (Stewart and Roter, 1989; Chewning and Sleath, 1996). This, it is argued, will produce the greatest health gain by combining active participation of the patient with the insights of a professional who is able to guide them through their options. Thus it can reduce problems with *non-compliance* associated with low patient input or possibly ill-informed choices when the clinician's skills are not utilized.

Table 7.1 Interaction between physician control and patient control

Physician control		
Patient control	Low	High
Low	Default	Paternalism
High	Consumerist	Mutuality

Undoubtedly this picture of collaborative endeavour between clinician and patient is attractive, but it requires a contribution from both parties to enable a suitably mature relationship to develop. Such an interaction can be jeopardized by either party. Clinicians cannot force patients to engage in this fashion, although there is some tantalising evidence to suggest that coaching patients in advance of their consultations might be highly effective (Kaplan *et al.*, 1989).

By default, most patients who are not using their treatment as the clinician intended are demonstrating a desire and capacity to exert control over the process. Thus it might be assumed that they would have a preference for an active role in any decisions about their care.

Case example

One businessman had a tense relationship with his family doctors because they did not trust him to manage his condition as much as he felt he could. Specifically, he wanted supplies of prednisolone and antibiotics for emergency use, but he did not engage with routine efforts to monitor his care. His desire for a consumerist relationship provoked a paternalistic response from his doctors, and a lack of trust in both directions resulted. By providing the emergency treatment that he sought, he was given greater control over and responsibility for his illness.

> Doctor: *"But for you what you really need is to be ... is to have the sort of power ... as much power as you can over your own drugs and stuff."*
> Patient: *"It's our destination, isn't it?"*
> Doctor: *"That's right."*
> Patient: *"I think in the modern day it should be a discussion. It shouldn't be a one-way discussion."*

In addition, this patient was keen to play down his asthma and disliked his inhalers – for instance, he never used them in public. It was thought that he was having difficulty fully accepting his condition. The improved therapeutic relationship allowed the implications of this to be discussed and education about treatment use and monitoring to be introduced. Some limits to treatment use could then be agreed and a more explicit agreement about sharing control negotiated.

Although control may not be the principal problem, it may facilitate a solution through renegotiating roles. During the process, some patients gain confidence and take more control – for instance, by assuming responsibility for monitoring hypertension. After discussion about the risk associated with untreated hypertension (to confirm that there is sufficient understanding to facilitate a testing period), a change of treatment is discussed and control over blood pressure monitoring is offered to this patient to help him to assess the value of treatment.

> Doctor: "I'll prescribe you another pill. Would you like you to try that, you know for a month, and come and see me? And if you want to take blood pressure readings at home before you come and see me that would probably be ..."
> Patient: "A better ... yes."
> Doctor: "The better way of doing it because you'd be convinced that it was a fair reflection of what your blood pressure was doing."
> Patient: "Yes, when I did it at home it seemed to soon settle down."

Acknowledging that doubts remain about the accuracy and role of home blood pressure monitoring, this approach at least included the patient in such a way that he chose to resume taking his treatment (Little et al., 2002).

Case example: Susan (continued)

> Let me use them when I feel I need them and not this morning. ... Not this four times a day. ... I know the tablets I must take, morning and night. And I know my morning inhalers, but during the day let me work it out when and if I need them; and if I need them, take them.

This extract has been cited to illustrate a patient who had insufficient confidence to be open about her medication use. It shows how she progressed during the intervention from being a passive, poorly informed and dangerously uncontrolled asthmatic, to a much more active patient whose clinical care improved dramatically.

Control has been considered relevant to treatment use for many years, but has not predicted *compliance* well (Calnan, 1989). However, apparent *compliance* could be expected from both passive and active patients, but for different reasons. Passive patients aim to 'comply', whereas active patients, who understand the treatment rationale sufficiently, elect to follow it appropriately.

Examples have been given of patients accepting more control, or at least more open control, over treatment, but also of patients who clearly state that they wish the doctor to retain control and be directive. Both situations were associated with an apparent clinical improvement, at least in the short term, indicating that some change resulted. Patients' level of control over their drugs should therefore be seen as open to negotiation and tailored to their need, but allowance has to be made for a reluctance to state this openly.

The question remains as to why some of these *non-compliant* patients, who were already demonstrating an 'active' behavior, should decline an invitation to take greater responsibility and control. Paradoxically, an empathic approach may engender greater trust in the practitioner, perhaps making patients happier to leave some decisions to their doctor without feeling the need to resist their advice. It has been claimed that patient-centered consultations increase *compliance*, and this increased trust is one potential mechanism for this (Stewart, 1995). Alternatively, clinicians may simply fail to adequately convey willingness for patients to make their own treatment choices and leave them trapped in a passive role. However, giving patients the option of making decisions may also be threatening, and could result in them wanting to retain a comfortable, passive role and follow advice once more. Such individuals might be expected to genuinely want to follow advice with regard to treatment, but may simply be unable to do so effectively. Although some 'tips and tricks' regarding recall and a supportive interaction may be sufficient, a more formal assessment of their motivation might be appropriate.

When clinicians feel that they are taking risks by providing treatment that patients request but which may not accord fully with accepted practice or guidelines, they can protect themselves by ensuring that patients are aware of any risks they are taking, and that this is documented. This issue is considered in more depth in Chapter 8.

Motivation

It can be tempting to assume that low motivation is the primary reason why many patients do not use their treatments in an effective manner. After all, provided that the benefits and use of treatment have been explained, why else would someone not want to follow advice that is offered in good faith? If this were the case, further information and *compliance* aids of various kinds would resolve the problem, which they clearly do not (Haynes *et al.*, 1996; Ebrahim, 1998). However, there are also individuals who understand the reasons for treatment, acknowledge their condition and have no apparent reason for not using treatment effectively, but just cannot manage to do so. It appears that these individuals have a problem with their motivation. Our experience suggests that these people often have substantial long-term health problems that eventually make them feel helpless and unable to achieve any real control over their health. As a consequence they give up. This may include giving up on their medicines as well as on other more onerous tasks, such as diet, as they come to feel that nothing has much effect.

This section acknowledges that this is a common issue in healthcare that relates to many problems such as diet, exercise and addictions. It is a most challenging task to instil motivation in someone else, and there is an entire literature and industry developing around this. There is no reason to think that medication use should be any more or less responsive, but a small number of consultations are not likely to achieve great progress unless they coincide with another substantial cue for behavior change.

Case example: Bill (continued)

Bill was in his mid-forties. He was grossly overweight, and had diabetes, cardiomyopathy and resulting atrial fibrillation. He was well aware of his increased risk of heart disease, and his ability to exercise was severely limited by his weight and shortness of breath. He was delighted to be invited for review, but it soon became apparent that he had given up on his health, was unable to maintain a healthy diet and consequently decided that taking his medication regularly was simply a waste of time. His problems appeared overwhelming to both him and his doctor, but he was happy to be directed towards positive steps that he could take. He did not want to become involved with decision making. After checking that he had a working understanding of his condition, that he accepted it and that he genuinely wanted the doctor to be in control, a goal was set to resume hypoglycaemic agents and commence swimming via an exercise-on-prescription scheme. The former proved possible, but the latter was thwarted by the fact that a large enough swimsuit was not available. Unfortunately, Bill collapsed and died a few months later.

Determining that motivation is a patient's primary difficulty is a process of exclusion. It may appear tempting to assume that this is the case because it avoids any inferred blame falling on clinical staff for providing ineffective explanations, or on patients for not adequately coming to terms with their diagnoses. However, it is probably the most complex problem to manage. Although a reinvigorated, more collaborative clinical relationship can precipitate a trial of treatment or challenge thinking, it is not a reliable way of motivating long-term behavior change. With such poorly motivated patients a directive counselling approach such as *motivational interviewing* may be ideal (Miller and Rollnick, 1991; Rollnick *et al.*, 1999). This more positive and structured approach appeared to be useful but was not assessed in our work, and is beyond the scope of this text. However, if you are interested you may wish to start by referring to *Health Behaviour Change* (Rollnick *et al.*, 1999).

Agree therapeutic goals

All of the consultation models, but especially those with an emphasis on shared decision making, suggest that it is helpful to conclude with a summary of specific actions that will be taken by each party and an agreement regarding follow-up. This is especially important if the treatment goals discussed or the intended treatment use vary from normal practice. Particular care should be taken to restate and record the patient's objectives, as these should be revisited at review, and may not be remembered or even considered at all if another clinician is involved. Acknowledging that each party has objectives helps to avoid the dominance of the medical agenda and reassures the patient that their values do count.

Conclusion

This chapter has argued that the process of successfully negotiating treatment use can vary from a simple rapidly achieved tacit agreement to a complex psychotherapeutic interaction. It is not necessary to invest time in formal decision-sharing approaches on all occasions, but in order to be effective clinicians should have the ability to do so when required. There are additional difficulties when managing established unhelpful patterns of medication use. These may require the clinician or the patient to adjust their stance before a resolution can be reached. This is entirely consistent with the principles of patient-centered prescribing as well as the more recent shift advocated in *From Compliance to Concordance* (Blenkinsopp *et al.*, 1997). Although a number of specific techniques have been suggested for understanding and managing these interactions effectively, by far the most important element is the clinician's value system. Only if the clinician genuinely believes that the patient has the right to determine their own choices will they be willing to create the environment that allows this to happen.

Chapter 8

Unresolved issues in patient-centered prescribing

Jon Dowell

Being realistic

This section will identify some of the unresolved issues that patients' and clinicians' rights, duties and responsibilities pose for those advocating this approach. These will be considered at an individual, professional and societal level. The potential conflict between clinical algorithms or guidelines and patient choice will be reintroduced along with a discussion of the potential legal pitfalls with this approach and suggestions about how practitioners may protect themselves from allegations of poor practice. Recent legal precedent from the UK will be used to support this. Additional special situations discussed will include when others are at risk, patient competency, manipulative patients and patients who wish to play a passive role.

There are a number of inherent conflicts in the process of prescribing medicines, and in many ways these are made more acute when seeking to be patient-centered. Many of these difficulties have been introduced or alluded to earlier in the book, but in this chapter each is presented and discussed in more depth. Where possible, practical examples are used for illustration, but because these issues are relatively rare, some are hypothetical rather than based on our experiences. Although suggestions are proffered for avoiding or managing some of the difficulties identified, these should be considered speculative, as this area of prescribing is developing rapidly and new ideas and precedents will no doubt develop.

The balance between the needs or preferences of the individual and clinicians' beliefs or societal role are at the root of most of the dilemmas presented below. Although human behaviors are probably universal, at least in most western contexts, the organization of healthcare varies considerably and in important ways across the globe. As the authors of this book are primarily based in the UK, some readers may be puzzled by consequences of the UK's National Health Service system which may not be so relevant to them, particularly in fee-paying or private systems or under different legal systems. Non-UK readers should therefore bear this in mind.

Part 1: Individual issues

Patient-centered prescribing, with its focus on tailoring the provision of medicines to the needs, beliefs and preferences of individual patients, challenges a number of the rules by which people normally operate. Some of these concern the roles that we tend to assume and the shift of power from clinician to patient that this process embodies. Clinicians' roles include some formal requirements, such as assessing individual patients' competence and seeking to apply accepted standards of practice, increasingly through the use of evidence-based guidelines. However, some personal traits and behavioral norms are also relevant here. In particular we shall discuss how clinicians and patients behave within consultations, and how patients' desire to exercise control over their care can vary and will affect their need for a patient-centered approach.

Behavioral norms for clinicians and patients

Clinical encounters in any healthcare context tend to develop fairly formulaic, predictable patterns. These will vary according to context – for example, a 'chat with a pharmacist' is distinct from consulting your family doctor, which is different again from a trip to an emergency room or casualty department. Most parties come to recognize the accepted rules for each encounter, and usually follow them quite closely. For instance, patients most commonly bring a problem which they expect to be asked to explain, and then usually would expect a treatment or advice to help them to resolve the problem. Traditionally there is also an expectation that the patient will value and follow the guidance given. These norms are very useful, as they are efficient (ground rules such as confidentiality do not need to be restated every time) and they facilitate exchange of intimate details and even touch that would not be acceptable outside this context. Professionals often spend considerable time during their training learning how to operate efficiently using these norms, and patients also consciously apply them during their healthcare encounters (Cromarty, 1996). A common approach is important, and probably has a considerable influence on resulting satisfaction and enablement. However, these norms also have drawbacks. For instance, they make it difficult for many patients to openly discuss the way they use or wish to use treatment, due to fear of courting criticism, jeopardising the clinical relationship or perhaps implying criticism of the prescriber.

The existing norms have developed over a long period, and they also take time and effort to change. As has been described in detail by Stewart *et al.* (2003), the shift towards a more balanced interaction requires a considerable shift away from the 'traditional' view of the medical encounter. Although many clinicians consider themselves to be practicing in a patient-centered manner, there is certainly considerable scope for a further shift, particularly in the so-called 'neglected second half of the consultation' (Elwyn *et al.*, 1999a) – the period in which treatment decisions are made, rather than information being gleaned from patients.

The development of a more collaborative approach requires new skills from both parties. Although this book is aimed at encouraging clinicians to develop their own skills, there is no doubt that more assertive patients assist this process (Kaplan *et al.*, 1989). Whatever skills participants may have, they also require a desire to operate in this manner. In particular, clinicians may be reluctant to include patients as fully as this process requires. Unless they are willing to share some of their existing authority, it requires a highly assertive patient and often a tense consultation for this to be wrested from them.

Case example

Here an unusually organized and assertive patient announces her agendas immediately on entering the consultation with a family doctor she knows well. Even the niceties of a welcome are skipped, and the tone is set for a consultation in which the patient participates very actively, in part due to the doctor's receptive response.

> Patient: *"So originally when I made the appointment it was only to see you about my HRT."*
> Doctor: *"Mm."*
> Patient: *"And to ask you a question about my eye, but I've taken this flu thing and I feel absolutely gubbed with it."*
> Doctor: *"OK. What do you want to deal with first?"*
> Patient: *"Right, the HRT, it's due in about, I think it's a week or a few days or whatever."*
> Doctor: *"You're on Premarin – any problems with it?"*

Of course these changes have implications for both parties. Patients will hopefully enjoy a greater say in their care, but they may also perceive the doctor as less decisive and may have less confidence in them. Likewise, clinicians may feel less competent when they have to perform the more complex and less scientific assimilation of patients' values with clinical decision making. Thus there appears to be a long way to go before most clinicians will wish to and be able to offer a patient-centered approach to prescribing for those who prefer this type of collaborative relationship. As Stewart and her colleagues advocate, this requires much more than a few skills that can be acquired with a little practice (Stewart *et al.*, 2003). It is an approach to practice that requires not only a range of skills, but also an underlying belief system that values individuals and their autonomy above professional ego or image. The same argument has been applied to the consent process for operative procedures, where it has also been suggested that there is a risk that we merely 'give a patient-centered veneer to disease-centered management' (Bridson *et al.*, 2003). Assuming that we want to, how can both patients and clinicians develop the skills required to change the culture of consultations?

The choice to be passive

In Chapter 5 we discussed how a patient's preferred role could be ascertained, and we suggested that this should be respected. So patients who do not wish to play a substantial role in deciding which treatment they receive should not be obliged to do so. Being patient-centered requires clinicians to make it simple for the patient to be as involved as they wish, not to force it upon them. Here we shall briefly revisit the issues that are raised by this as they relate to the common consultation behavior patterns outlined above.

There is evidence that some patients prefer and are helped by a doctor who has a directive style. For instance, Thomas (1987, 1994) found that a practitioner with a confident and directive style had an even greater benefit for non-specific minor infections than the use of a placebo tablet. Many doctors believe that it is best to appear confident and decisive in order to appear competent. There is also evidence that most patients prefer doctors to dress in a formal way, perhaps to reinforce the expected authority of the role (McKinstry and Wang, 1991). There is therefore conflict between studies which show that patient involvement, as advocated by patient-centered medicine, is beneficial, and some evidence and a common belief that employing a decisive style has merits. The solution is surely to recognize that patients differ and that their needs will vary depending on the nature of their problem and situation. During acute, critical events even the most assertive, articulate individual is unlikely to want to discuss their options in detail. They are vulnerable, have little autonomy, and are likely to feel relieved if they can simply place trust in their carers (Tobias and Souhami, 1993). However, the same individual may wish to be well informed and fully involved in decisions about long-term treatments such as antihypertensive agents or anticoagulants. Indeed they may well simply not accept advice or treatment if they don't feel that their views have been considered. There are a variety of different types of patient, and their preferences will change depending on the situation. The challenge for clinicians is to be able to offer a range of styles of decision making and also to be able to assess which is most appropriate during any one consultation, rather than simply applying their preferred approach on all occasions.

However, it is important to remember that each party's role does not start from scratch. Even in a first consultation about a new condition, the powerful traditions that govern expected and normally acceptable roles within medical encounters immediately come into play. Consequently, clinicians who commence consultations with a traditional style, even if they are genuinely willing and able to change their style, will have begun by reinforcing the prevailing model of interaction, and made their patient feel less involved and less likely to openly discuss *non-compliance*. Patient-centered prescribing therefore requires a shift from the outset in order to set a more collaborative tone for the encounter that will encourage and empower the patient to be candid about their views and planned or actual behavior. It cannot be tagged on to a disease-centered interaction as an afterthought.

Even recent studies of doctor–patient interactions suggest that the historical power imbalance persists, and that doctors still rarely actively involve patients in treatment decisions (Tuckett *et al.*, 1985; Byrne and Long, 1989; Stevenson *et al.*, 2000; Elwyn *et al.*, 2003). As many patients will have had little or no experience of being actively involved in treatment decisions, it is perhaps not surprising that the status quo is only changing slowly, and that patient demand is only increasing gradually. The question is therefore not when patients should be involved, but why it is not standard practice, when it is not appropriate, and how clinicians can find out.

How can clinicians establish what role patients wish to play in deciding about treatment? Undoubtedly this remains an inexact process, and it must always rely heavily on the subtleties of interpersonal communication and a sound relationship. Because of the long history of paternalistic medical practice, the balance should be addressed by starting with a patient-centered approach, and only revert to a traditional style cautiously.

Evidence-based vs. individual care

In Chapter 2 it was suggested that the application of data from clinical trials to individual care should be considered critically. Sometimes evidence-based medicine

(EBM) is presented as incompatible with patient choice and therefore patient-centered care, but this is a narrow-minded approach. Although we should realize the limitations of EBM, we should not disregard its value. Instead we should seek to intelligently use the condensation of evidence that it provides to help patients to make sensible choices for themselves. EBM can help to better inform patients as well as clinicians. It is up to us to help them to use this information.

It has been suggested that interventions can be broadly categorized as *effective* (where benefits are known to be large compared with harms) and *preference sensitive* (where the ratio of benefit to harm is uncertain or dependent upon patient preferences) (O'Connor *et al.*, 2003b). As the evidence becomes weaker or more finely balanced, some would see patient choice as becoming more legitimate. Here we shall consider the difficulty of balancing 'the evidence' (strong or weak) against the principle of being patient-centered in approach.

Whether considering individual studies, evidence-based practice or clinical guidelines, the statistical interpretation of findings is based upon sampling representative populations of subjects. We cannot know whether the individual considering treatment will be fortunate and benefit from therapy, or unfortunate and suffer side-effects, or both. Unless the treatment is purely symptomatic, we can probably never know, and must simply consider each patient as 'average.' This problem of assuming an individual's response based on the results of clinical trials has been termed the 'clinical evidence gap', and has caused eminent researchers to state that 'clinical trials are the best way to assess what interventions work, but the worst way to assess who will benefit' (Mant, 1999). Perhaps the 'n of 1' trial will become common practice in the future, but for now we may need to more formally try things out *with* patients rather than *on* them (March, 1994).

Most studies and guidelines are developed exclusively on the basis of clinical outcomes such as reduced blood pressure or occurrence of stroke, rather than patient preference data. Clearly the former will often reflect the latter, but this is not necessarily so. Again, individual patients will have different values – although, unlike their physiological response to treatments, their values are accessible through discussion. Thus it should be possible to tailor therapeutic advice to the individual patient's beliefs and values. For instance, a hypertensive patient would be advised to reduce their blood pressure primarily in order to reduce the risk of a stroke, commonly by using an antihypertensive treatment. However, in order to avoid one event it is often necessary to treat many hundreds of patients (the numbers needed to treat depending upon the individual's risk profile). Most patients will not benefit from treatment, yet many will suffer some side-effects, while others will dislike the idea of actually taking treatment (Benson and Britten, 2002). The potential cost to the patient of the latter component can only be accessed through discussion at the time when therapeutic decisions are being made.

Guidelines and EBM usually focus on the management of a single condition, whereas, especially with aging populations, clinicians are often dealing with multiple problems, and both patient and clinician may have justifiable concerns about problems arising from the resulting polypharmacy.

Guidelines reflect 'best' care as a way of summarising an overwhelming volume of research data. They deliberately simplify advice that is limited to the principal recognized groups of patients. They assist clinicians in tailoring treatment, but only crudely. We must also acknowledge that the data on which they are based are often imperfect in terms of their limited statistical power, as well as concerns remaining about the robustness of most research findings. Thus guidelines may be the best we have available at present, but they are not perfect. Current research is focussing on decision support techniques, especially using computer-based systems that allow patients' values to be included, but these are not yet commonly available, and they seem to have surprisingly little effect on the eventual outcome (Montgomery *et al.*, 2003).

There is overwhelming evidence that clinicians find systematically applying guidelines difficult in practice (Grimshaw and Russell, 1993). Primarily this appears to be because they find it difficult to alter their existing working practices, rather than because patients are reluctant to accept guideline-based advice (Davis and Thomson, 1995; Cabana *et al.*, 1999; Premaratne *et al.*, 1999; Rousseau, 2003). In many ways this difficulty with building evidence-based guidelines into clinical practice has parallels with the process of patient-centered prescribing. Doctors commonly express scepticism about guidelines, and complain that they limit their 'clinical freedom' and patients appear no better at complying with such guidance than do patients with prescribed drugs. Clinicians seem not to intuitively take to guidelines, much as patients tend to 'not take medicines unless I have to.'

The rigid adherence to any evidence base, ahead of the views of a competent patient, is contrary to the spirit of patient-centered medical care. Although guidelines do assimilate evidence efficiently and make this available at the point of patient contact, which is an essential service, it is not a sufficient solution. Many guideline proponents who also advocate including patient preferences and choice do acknowledge this. There is no philosophical conflict between high-quality evidence being used and care being centered on the patient (Stewart *et al.*, 2003). It is how this is done that presents the difficulty (Bridson *et al.*, 2003).

An unfortunate by-product of the evidence-based shift in medicine is that clinicians find it difficult to advocate treatments that do not follow what are becoming increasingly established guidelines. This may be a good thing, as an increasing proportion of treatment becomes standardized and effective. However, it is problematic if this is done at the expense of patient preference, not least because this is likely to result in reduced *compliance*. Clinicians may feel more confident defending their actions if they can say 'I told them to take drug X, as per these guidelines', rather than 'We discussed this and agreed that drug Y was preferable for them even though it's not so effective (or the cheapest or the first choice, etc.).' The barrier that this defensive approach presents must be addressed before patient-centered therapeutic decision making can become the norm in any area of medicine. In the UK, at least, the legal situation remains in favour of patient choice, and the clinician can adequately protect him- or herself from litigation with appropriate note keeping. This is discussed in more detail below. However, there may also be other pressures to conform to prescribing guidelines that are principally driven by cost. Financial incentives or other pressures may be used to induce clinicians to prescribe 'rationally.' From a societal perspective this may make good sense. However, on an individual basis it may limit choice, and clinicians may need to be open about the pressures that the healthcare system exerts on them. There is evidence that patients are willing to accept these financial constraints if they are asked appropriately (Dowell *et al.*, 1996).

Ethical and legal dilemmas: competence ar consent

In the UK, General Medical Council ethical guidelines emphasize that all adu have the authority to decline treatment, even if the health of another, su unborn child, may be affected (General Medical Council, 2002). These guidelin_ _.lect the legal situation in the UK. The British courts have made it clear that an adult patient who is mentally competent has the right to make his or her own healthcare decisions, even where these decisions conflict with medical advice (reported in 1992, *All England Reports*, Vol. 4, p. 649). The judge in that case stated:

> An adult patient who suffers from no mental incapacity has an absolute right to choose whether to consent to medical treatment, to refuse it or to choose one rather than another of the treatments being offered.

However, in order to do so the patient needs to be informed, which is the clinician's responsibility. But how far does this responsibility extend? This was tested recently in the English High Court (Unreported case: *T Kent v Griffiths v Others*. High Court, The Strand, London, July 1999). The patient suffered from asthma and had been taking inhaled steroids to manage her condition. When she became pregnant, she was worried about the adverse effects that the medication might have on her unborn child, and decided to stop taking her medication. Her asthma worsened, so she consulted her family doctor, who confirmed that her peak-flow measurement was reduced. She asked for a prescription for salbutamol, which she was given, and her doctor advised her to start taking steroids once more. Still troubled by her asthma, she consulted a second time and was again advised to resume her steroid inhaler. She chose not to follow this advice, and suffered a severe asthma attack 5 days later that caused her to miscarry and to suffer profound amnesia. The patient thereafter sued the doctors involved, claiming that she ought to have been given stronger advice about the dangers of her decision. However, the judge concluded that the doctors had not been negligent because they had twice recorded advice to resume steroids, were able to demonstrate consistently high-quality care for asthmatic patients, and explained why it was not their normal practice to 'scare patients' into using medicines. Although reassuring, this case does raise issues about the level of information required to support an 'informed' or 'shared' decision, and how practitioners can defend such discussions about risk.

In order to fulfil their duty of care, doctors should give their advice, including the likely severity of the consequences of not following it. For a legal defence these details should be documented.

These legal precedents also require the patient to be 'competent' to make their own judgements, in what might reasonably be considered 'a sound mind.' The subtlety of these distinctions is illustrated by the case of a 68-year-old schizophrenic man who developed gangrene in one foot (*Adult: refusal of medical treatment*. Reported in 1994, *All England Reports*, Vol. 1, p. 819). His doctors wanted to amputate his leg below the knee, and predicted that his chances of surviving without such an operation were only 15%. The patient refused the operation and was granted an injunction preventing the hospital from carrying out the operation without his written consent. The court judged that during lucid intervals the patient was capable of making his own medical decisions, and was entitled to refuse treatment. So how is a patient's 'competence' to make decisions about healthcare determined, and when might it be appropriate to question this? Commonly this is a simple and brief consideration, but not always. This case demonstrates that the distinction between competence and incompetence may be a fine one.

Most of these legal cases have been brought to resolve acute, 'one-off' decisions regarding surgery, transfusions, etc., and not ongoing medication that requires the active participation of the individual. Unless in residential care, it is hard to imagine how medication use could be enforced against someone's will. So in the vast majority of cases the patient's active consent is a prerequisite for any successful pharmacological treatment, and it is contrary to the law, as well as paternalistic, not to ensure that informed consent is obtained. Although this can be – and often is – assumed, this is not so when dissent has been implied by *non-compliance*.

Patients who make 'inappropriate' requests or are manipulative

There is a small but time-consuming group of patients who seek clearly inappropriate treatment, or who seek treatment in inappropriate ways. Here we would include those who seek drugs of abuse or who pressure doctors to prescribe unnecessary treatment, and the few who relate inappropriately to the clinician. For instance, a patient with a cold or flu-like illness might, in the UK context, threaten to 'just get the doctor out tonight if it's not better' in response to a clinician who does not believe that antibiotics are a suitable treatment.

It is difficult to create a collaborative therapeutic relationship quickly in these situations, and attempting to engage the patient in a more constructive relationship by the application of patient-centered approaches as advocated in this book or other texts may not suffice (Elwyn *et al.*, 1999b; Stewart *et al.*, 2003). We must acknowledge that there are occasions when attending to building the relationship, providing time and understanding the patient's perspective do not lead to a comfortable resolution. There is not always sufficient time available to manage these situations ideally. The clinician can either acquiesce (which risks encouraging this type of manipulative or even threatening approach) or decline (which risks provoking resentment or even anger and further calls out of hours). Resolving such outright conflicts is not the focus of this book, but readers may wish to refer to *Skills for Communicating with Patients* (Silverman *et al.*, 1998, p. 124) or *Getting to Yes* (Fisher *et al.*, 1992). Those authors suggest attempting to separate the position (antibiotics or not) from the interests ('I need to get better as soon as possible' vs. 'I want to prescribe rationally') and thereby create an opportunity for discussing other mutually acceptable outcomes. This may require time, delicate negotiating skills and compromises such as the use of so-called 'delayed prescribing' (when patients are issued a prescription to meet their expectations, but asked to await events for an agreed time to see whether the symptoms begin to resolve spontaneously). On some occasions there may be insufficient common ground and it becomes necessary to fall back on your 'next best option' to a mutually acceptable solution. For instance, you may conclude that the risks and cost of providing an antibiotic for a viral infection do not justify jeopardising a sound clinical relationship, and therefore you may acquiesce. By contrast, you might prefer that a drug addict is frustrated or irritated rather than perpetuate unacceptable demands for drugs of abuse. Recognising your 'bottom line' in advance is helpful, but should not prevent attempts to move beyond the initial conflict. If the primary conflict can be set aside, many of the strategies outlined in Chapter 6 are likely to be useful for achieving a mutually acceptable compromise, especially those aimed at managing *non-compliant* patients where there is often an element of conflict, either implied or explicit. By sidestepping rather than confronting the main barrier (whether it is an unreasonable request or hidden *non-compliance*), an opportunity is sought to establish common ground which can be built upon. Often this is a desirable therapeutic goal for both parties and, working backwards from this, a more acceptable solution may be sought.

Getting out of depth

When deliberately seeking to establish more trusting, stronger therapeutic relationships with patients who are perceived to be in special need of such a bond, clinicians are likely to emphasize their empathic responses and use other gestures to demonstrate that they care (Balint, 1964). As a result, it is more likely that substantial and possibly new emotive issues may be raised. These attempts to 'connect' may be misinterpreted by some patients, particularly those who are lonely, or who have learning disabilities or mental health problems. Therefore practitioners should be capable of stepping back and considering the process, recognising when progress cannot be made or even when an unhelpful dependence may be created. McWhinney (1989) suggests that identifying this and being familiar with steps to disengage are particularly important when employing patient-centered approaches.

Case example: Paul

Paul was 40 years old, had mild learning difficulties, lived alone and required regular medication. His treatment use was chaotic, and in desperation his doctors arranged for him to attend the surgery daily for this. He complied with this arrangement. After being invited to discuss his situation using the techniques described in Chapter 6, he quickly started to reveal details of abuse and to seek frequent appointments for trivial reasons. Once formal counselling was established, the doctor attempted to reduce the frequency of appointments, which provoked episodes of minor self-harm to justify further reviews. Gradually it was possible to establish a more satisfactory pattern of weekly reviews and minimal intervening urgent consultations.

Although this might be regarded as a success in some ways, it required considerable time and emotional energy. We might conclude that there are a few patients for whom concordant therapeutic decisions are never going to be achieved, and other cases where clinicians may not even wish to try. However, this should not stop us trying for those who are likely to benefit.

In this section we have considered specific difficulties that can arise during consultations when trying to prescribe in a patient-centered manner. We now move on to examine what professional and inter-professional issues also need to be considered. Increasingly, the ways in which professionals interrelate are being seen as an important component of the care process, and this so-called 'relationship-centered' approach to the whole care package is important for patient-centered prescribing as well as more acute team situations, such as resuscitation (Gittel, 2003).

Part 2: Professional issues

Changing working practices have implications for professionals, who must adapt their own behaviors. These adaptations are driven by and therefore related to the key driving forces behind the process. So, for instance, a shift towards patient-centered prescribing might sometimes specifically require more discussion time with patients, different record-keeping practices and greater collaborative working with colleagues across different professions. These practical issues reflect the broader forces of change and represent the mechanisms by which they are brought about. They are discussed here in purely practical terms, although they link to the underlying issues that are discussed in the sections both above and below. However, these practical details are of key importance to clinical staff, and can have a huge effect on the degree of success. Clinicians must be able to reconcile the various pressures on their time, resources and skills satisfactorily or they will not be able to maintain any change in service.

Time requirements

Whatever the resources available to healthcare systems, throughout the world clinicians universally appear to consider themselves short of time. Any change that might demand an additional time investment is likely to be resisted. There are two potential responses to this. First, it might be possible to use the existing time to greater effect by incorporating new consulting techniques. This argument has been used to support being patient-centered in general, and there are a number of studies which suggest that skilled patient-centered consulters can achieve greater success without requiring longer consultations (Stewart *et al.*, 2003). It seems likely that the techniques advocated for patient-centered consulting are intrinsically more efficient than a traditional history-taking approach, especially in the primary care setting (Silverman *et al.*, 1998). Secondly, as clinicians currently rarely provide patients with the information that they require in order to engage in treatment decisions, it is difficult to see how this can be done without some additional time. There are three ways in which this might be countered.

1 It can be argued that involving patients from the outset should reduce future return visits due to greater commitment to treatment and hence condition control, so there may be no greater time demand in the longer term.
2 If patient care is improved, extra time invested may be justified. If surgeons rushed operations and produced poor outcomes, this would not be considered appropriate. Why should the prescribing process not be considered from this perspective? How long should it take to gain a commitment to lifelong therapy?
3 Both of these arguments are particularly pertinent when managing patients whose conditions are poorly controlled due to their suboptimal use of medications. These individuals are demonstrating their desire to be involved more in decisions about their treatment in a very pragmatic way, by not *complying*. Time spent with them is especially likely to result in improved care and therefore reduced future morbidity. The case of Susan (introduced in Chapter 2) illustrates this well.
4 There may be an increasing expectation, demand and even moral argument that it is the clinician's responsibility to ensure that patients are informed about and thereby able to consent fully to their therapies. We no longer live in the 'Trust me I'm a

doctor' age, and this may be a required progression for western medicine as it seeks to retain its pre-eminence as the dominant healing paradigm. In the UK at least, it is clear that quality of care is related to consultation length, and there is an increasing demand for systematic changes that encourage less rushed interactions (Freeman *et al.*, 2002) and increasing patient involvement.

Inter-professional working

Clinical care is gradually becoming more of a team activity in many different ways. Specialist doctors, generalists and nurse practitioners of different kinds are increasingly sharing patient care using a myriad of protocols, guidelines and informal local networks. How can such systems accommodate to include patients' preferences as has been described in this book? One answer, of course, is that they already do for some individuals, usually those who have already found it beneficial to take a very active role in their care. These individuals are able to act as their own advocates. The problem is that discussion with one clinician which results in agreeing to a 'non-standard' approach is not time well spent if this discussion is repeated or ignored by other clinicians. We cannot claim to have any clever solutions to this issue, but seek to highlight it and trust that sensitive clinicians will listen to patients' accounts of how they made such decisions, and respect their patients' and their colleagues' approach. Perhaps the way in which we view 'continuity of care' needs to evolve for this to happen. Continuity of 'philosophy of care' or relationship style rather than care given may assist this, and will hopefully be aided by changes in record-keeping practice as discussed below.

Information and understanding

As well as having capacity to consent to treatment, a patient must have the requisite information, and be able to understand that information, before responsibility for decisions can be handed over. Thus clinicians must ensure that they give patients adequate information about the potential risks and benefits of treatment, as well as details of suitable alternatives, including no action at all. Clinicians should also check that the patient understands these risks. For example, the schizophrenic patient with a gangrenous leg (cited earlier in this chapter) had been informed about his likely prognosis should an amputation not be performed, and it was deemed that he had understood he might die. In contrast, when Mrs T, a Jehovah's Witness who had initially signed to refuse blood transfusion, deteriorated unexpectedly the court felt she may not initially have fully understood the consequences of refusal. While the court emphasised the principle of patient autonomy, it found she had not been able to make a sufficiently informed decision (reported in 1992, *All England Reports*, Vol 4, p.649).

There are a number of techniques that can be used to assist the efficient transfer of information that also help the clinician to appraise the recipient's understanding (Silverman *et al.*, 1998). In order to prescribe in a patient-centered manner it is important not only to be able to transfer information effectively, but also to aim to provide it in a balanced manner. This is a much more sophisticated skill than explaining how often a particular therapy should be taken. For instance, it may include deciding to emphasize a particular risk (of therapy or of the condition) because the patient had not appreciated it fully. They appeared not to have understood. This is not the same as framing or exaggerating the risk in order to convince the patient to do what the clinician might consider to be the best thing.

The standard that clinicians must reach if they are to avoid negligence claims in the UK was specified in 1957 – a clinician's actions will not be considered to have been negligent if they conformed to a practice which was accepted by a responsible body of medical opinion (1957, *All England Reports,* Vol. 2, p. 118). However, it should be noted that the judge in that case stated:

> A judge might, in certain circumstances, come to the conclusion that the disclosure of a particular risk was *so obviously necessary* to an informed choice on the part of the patient that no reasonably prudent doctor would fail to make it. *(my italics)*

This suggests that some risks are so important that all patients ought to be told about them. However, there may be a fine line between this and pressuring patients to accept treatment against their will – a situation that is contrary to the spirit of shared decision making and likely to result in *non-compliance*.

This process of providing information, checking understanding and when necessary recording the details of the discussion is key to the process of handing over responsibility to competent patients. The key components of record keeping will be discussed next.

Record keeping and handing over responsibility

Record keeping has four main roles. It assists recall of events, it enables audit of care, it provides communication between colleagues and, when necessary, it provides evidence in cases of litigation. It is the last two of these functions that we shall consider here, as they are relevant to inter-professional working and information provision as discussed above.

Clinical records provide an essential link between different episodes of care and different clinicians in both hospital and general practice, but they tend to be highly abridged records of interactions and are commonly very tightly focussed on the clinical details. Rarely is space given for the patient's beliefs or views about treatment. However, when the patient's perspective substantially changes the resulting treatment, it becomes as important to document their views as it would be to document any major examination finding. Consequently it is necessary to develop conventions for recording the patient's views efficiently and explicitly. This will help to prevent different clinicians revisiting decisions again and again, and is increasingly important the further away from established treatment the patient decides to go.

Clinicians must feel confident to help patients to reach their own decisions, but they can only do so if they also feel adequately protected professionally. Otherwise they will be tempted to cajole or pressure patients to accept the normal treatment. To encourage professionals to play an appropriate, balanced role, they require a mechanism to protect themselves from potential litigation. Although this sounds very defensive, clinicians require these precautions to enable true shared decision making to become normal practice. Otherwise it may be seen as a high-risk way to practice. Such defensive record keeping is only likely to be required on an occasional basis, as the majority of patients are always likely to accept a fairly standard, recommended treatment.

The key features of any defence should include the fact that inadequate information or warnings about potential adverse outcomes had been understood, and that it was the patient's decision to follow the course they did. Clearly both depend upon recording adequate details of the discussion. This includes summary details of the information given, and preferably a note that they were perceived to have understood any additional risks. In extreme circumstances it may be useful to symbolize this transfer of responsibility by asking the patient to sign the clinical notes as a 'disclaimer.' This ensures that the patient has acknowledged the implications, and allows the clinician to concentrate on providing care rather than worrying about litigation. Although verbal consent to or refusal of treatment is, strictly speaking, as valid in law as written consent, a patient's signature is good evidence that the conversation took place, and that the patient was indeed aware of the relevant information. Occasional experience of doing this suggests that the act of signing such a disclaimer brings home the seriousness of the decision and makes the patient pause to reconsider the risk in question. Such disclaimers ought to state that the patient has discussed their condition/options with the clinician, and has been made aware of the associated risks (not simply that they are 'going against medical advice'). Ideally, these risks should be stated, so that the nature and strength of the advice given by the clinician is made clear, but many may be wary of this step. The purpose of suggesting such an apparently draconian step is not to give rise to confrontation but to reduce it.

One other aspect of managing responsibility also needs to be considered. As more professions become involved in the prescribing process, particularly pharmacists and nurses, it is important to reflect on how they may become involved in this process. They commonly operate much more strictly according to protocols than doctors do, and they may feel a greater threat when deviating from those protocols. They are also often operating under various forms of delegated authority, and the responsible clinician must be confident that they are able to inform patients and share decisions effectively before they can practice in such a flexible, patient-centered way. When they do so, the decisions that they make with patients should be respected and not subsequently overruled by a paternalistic doctor. When they do not have such skills or flexibility, they should be encouraged to pass these decisions on rather than insist on a rigid protocol if they recognise that the patient does not support this.

We have now addressed a number of issues that may arise during the consultations in which patient-centered prescribing is being practiced, and considered how it may also require some changes in inter-professional working practices. However, the shift towards more patient-centered care and prescribing in particular also raises some issues for the societies in which we live and work. These will be considered below.

Part 3: Societal issues

So far we have primarily described patient-centered prescribing as being founded upon individuals having the ability to exercise their right to make choices between the options offered as potentially suitable. The clinician's expertise allows them to select which options are potentially suitable, rather than the patient. However, so far patient competency is the only limitation we have discussed.

Here we shall consider the balance that must be struck between the personal freedoms that all patient-centered approaches seek to enhance, and the potential societal costs that may result. All comprehensive healthcare systems have limited resources, and expenditure on medications will to some extent limit provision of other services or facilities. It must be acknowledged that patient-centered prescribing does not exist in isolation, and it should not be taken to mean that any competent patient should receive whatever treatments they want, whenever they want, and for whatever reason.

Patients who make 'unreasonable' requests

To what extent is it acceptable for patients to request therapy that is more expensive (e.g. a branded medicine rather than a generic one) or a therapy that has borderline or unknown efficacy? If the clinician's only duty was to that patient, then almost any prescribing could be justified on the basis that some benefit may result, placebo or otherwise, and that the therapeutic relationship may be protected by doing this. However, most clinicians would feel uncomfortable about this approach for at least two reasons. First, many would be concerned that unhelpful patterns of healthcare use might increase as a result. Secondly, most are aware of a need to distribute resources at least effectively, and possibly equitably as well. Such prescribing may be more acceptable in systems where patients fund their own treatments, and this includes the CAM therapies, where evidence may be weak or lacking (Coulter, 2003). It may also be more common in fee-for-service systems where there may be an incentive to generate further consultations. In contrast, under a universal state healthcare system there will be greater pressures and regulation to ration resource use efficiently.

Case example

A few years ago a female patient joined one of our practices, having moved into the area. She had suffered from low mood on and off for many years, but found conventional antidepressants either ineffective or intolerable. As a result of her own reading, she had previously requested, tried and come to believe in two unconventional therapies. Her previous family doctor had prescribed, at her request, selegiline and hydergine for depression and prevention of Alzheimer's disease. When she requested these medicines from her new doctor, he felt uncomfortable prescribing them, and sought guidance from the literature (including two Cochrane reviews) and a local consultant psychiatrist. Both indicated that there was no substantial evidence that these treatments were effective, yet they were expensive. What should the clinician do?

The more extravagant or therapeutically unreasonable a request is, the heavier the clinician's societal role is likely to weigh. Of course, the authority that is vested in the prescriber always allows such requests to be refused. This is the prescriber's choice and is the root of much power, but they must balance the immediate pressures of an insistent patient with a more abstract belief or value system with regard to their role. To what extent should they guard society's resources in the interests of equity and cost-effectiveness? Or in a private system, to what extent should they sanction treatments that may be ineffective or have greater risks than the conventional or evidence-based recommendation? Again, of course, we must acknowledge that there are weaknesses in the existing evidence base as well as in patients' beliefs. The potential effect of refusal on the clinical relationship is also very difficult to predict. This balance is summarized in the table below.

Factors that impinge on patient choice

Factors that favour patient choice	Factors that limit patient choice
Strong patient beliefs (based on research, anecdote or personal experience)	Strong clinicians beliefs (scientific evidence suggests better alternatives or lack of effect)
Insecure clinician (not sure of evidence or overeager to please patient)	Paternalistic clinician, irritation due to patient's approach
Low cost of patient's choice (or patient funded)	High cost of patient's choice
Low risk (of side-effects or lack of therapeutic effect)	High risk of potential harm
Close to usual practice (e.g. branded vs. generic product)	Very atypical practice (unlicensed use)
Patient accepting responsibility	Patient requires implied approval

These types of issues cannot be satisfactorily answered in general terms, as the context is usually crucial. However, the above table may help to clarify the components that clinicians might consider when faced with a difficult situation. Decisions will depend not only on the patient and the treatment being considered, but also on the healthcare system and professional norms that prevail at the time and place in question.

When others are at risk

Accepting and acting according to the patient's beliefs and choices becomes much more challenging if others are at risk as a result. Examples of this include treatment for pulmonary tuberculosis or HIV, or during pregnancy. In such situations the clinician may perceive, and sometimes has, a duty to protect others. The legal situation is not always clear, and precedents include a mother being allowed to decline a Caesarean section despite significant risk to the fetus (in the UK), and *non-compliant* tuberculosis patients being incarcerated for medical treatment (in the USA).

Compulsory medical treatment is extremely uncommon outside the mental health arena, and is likely to require court proceedings to ensure that human rights are preserved. Consequently, even when there is a risk to others, be it from tuberculosis or passive smoking in the home, there is little that clinicians can do apart from attempting to establish a relationship that facilitates patient information and thereby encourages them to reconsider their situation. There may be a justifiable moral case for pressuring a patient in this situation – for instance, by presenting risk information in a stark way – but a practical limitation in that this can simply engender resistance and entrench the position more deeply (Miller and Rollnick, 1991). There is some evidence that even tuberculosis in the developing world context is most effectively managed using purely collaborative approaches, and current understanding about inducing health behavior change suggests that poorly timed pressure will be counterproductive (Rollnick *et al.*, 1999; Maher *et al.*, 2003). Thus although clinicians may feel particularly impotent on such occasions, there is commonly little they can practically do. This may be another occasion when investing appreciable time, effort and skill in involving an unwilling partner in a collaborative process may be worthwhile.

Conclusion

This chapter has sought to identify and analyse some of the unresolved issues that may arise from the prescribing process when using a patient-centered approach. The balance between patients' and clinicians' rights and responsibilities is occasionally defined in law but must frequently be set in practice. The key difficulty arises when a patient selects an option or uses a treatment in such a way that they are exposed to an additional risk. For patient-centered prescribing to work, clinicians must feel free to enable such informed choices and to do so without accusations of malpractice. Ensuring high-quality record keeping, and if necessary asking patients to sign these records, should release clinicians from the threat of such accusations sufficiently for this to happen.

Chapter 9

Summary

Jon Dowell

This chapter seeks to review the core messages that we have tried to convey and put them into context with regard to the broader patient-centered approach. We also briefly touch upon suggestions for future areas of research.

Key aspects of patient-centered prescribing

Patient-centered prescribing is an evolving approach to the most common therapeutic action in western medicine. It continues a paradigm shift that is already well under way from the more traditional, so-called 'paternalistic' approach towards a collaborative interaction that is focussed on a therapeutic relationship and the patient's values. So in essence we are describing the need for partnerships and the complexities of achieving these when the clinician and the patient may not see eye to eye. As with other aspects of patient-centered medicine, this is as much about attitude and approach as it is about specific skills, so we make no apologies that some of the specific skills presented here may have appeared short on detail, be inadequately described or only weakly justified. This is a rapidly developing field, and we have repeatedly stated that we offer suggestions for improvement, not definitive solutions. Rather than focussing heavily on micro-skills, we invite you to consider whether the whole package might not have greater potential than the sum of its parts.

Patient-centered medicine has evolved and been refined over the last 20 years, which has affected the thinking behind as well as the practice of medicine throughout the western world. Having been increasingly widely applied, particularly to the diagnostic component of the interview, this approach is now reaching the closing stages – the 'neglected second half of the consultation' (Elwyn *et al.*, 1999a). The recognition that the care process does not benefit from the separation of feelings and thinking, or art and science, is being extended into the decisions made about treatment, the traditional domain of the professional. With confidence derived from growing evidence of benefits for both patients and clinicians, demonstrable success in teaching methods and parallel shifts in society's view of medicine, this philosophy (patient-centered medicine) is challenging the fundamental question of 'who knows best what is good for the patient.'

Whether driven by ethical arguments in favour of autonomy, or practical factors such as ineffective medication use and increasingly informed patients, there is no doubt that clinicians are learning to share information, decisions and responsibility better. Some professionals may perceive this as a threat, but it need not be so. Rather, it offers a chance to combine the benefits of medical expertise with patients' 'expertise in their person' to maximize the therapeutic value of the available treatments. It also offers some hope of resolution to the *compliance* 'problem.' Not only does it offer a pragmatic and principled approach for handling *non-compliance* in clinical practice, but it also reframes the 'problem' itself. *Compliance* with the clinician's instructions is no longer the goal. It need not be due to a failure of the clinician that someone makes apparently unhealthy choices or fails to successfully implement the treatment plans that they have agreed. Patient power is matched here with responsibility.

There are two innovative elements of this book that deserve to be highlighted at this point. First, we have attempted to combine pertinent behavioral and consultation models into a theoretically informed approach to help clinicians both to conceptualize and to apply patient-centered prescribing in practice. This should help to demystify the decision-sharing process and indicate how it can vary from very rapid, obvious decisions to repeated rounds of testing and reviewing. We have elected to use diagrams to illustrate our approach, not only because they aid understanding but also because they assist in predicting subsequent steps and help to identify areas that have been omitted. We recognize that they can give a false impression of a neat and ordered progression that we do not intend. The reality, of course, is that these interactions are complex and disorderly discussions, flitting from values to feelings, beliefs to experiences, and implicit to explicit forms of communication. Clearly one size does not fit all, and empathic support might hold the key for one, while an explicit treatment test or explanation of the disease might hold the key for others. A flexible approach in a spirit of partnership is advocated.

We then reported our experiences of attempting to achieve partnerships of this kind under the testing conditions presented by established *non-compliance*. Coping with the implied existing discord and lack of partnership is challenging, but offers an opportunity to make progress in what are clearly ineffective therapeutic relationships. Additional time and skills may be required to achieve this, but the principles remain the same. Stewart, her colleagues and others continue to amass persuasive evidence that patient-centered care is not only noticed by patients but also associated with greater satisfaction, reduced investigation and improved outcomes (Stewart *et al.*, 2003). In general, these studies have been conducted on whole populations of patients (e.g. in family practice or with breast cancer). It seems likely that focussing effort where the therapeutic partnership is weak is likely to be especially worthwhile and a realistic way to put 'concordance' into practice.

For practicing clinicians, we hope that this book taps into an existing desire to practice medicine using a patient-centered approach. From this position it is not a large jump to deliberately consider medication use and experiences from the patient's perspective in just the same way as their other beliefs and expectations are drawn into the melting pot. The sociological and psychological explanations for behavior given in Chapters 3 and 4 provide a framework within which to interpret these accounts and suggest interventions that might bring about a behavior change. The consultation model and techniques described in Chapters 6 and 7 should help you to envisage how this might be applied within your daily practice and when you elect to invest some extra effort to explore a patient's ineffective use of medication. However, there are a number of traps for the unwary and, as with other consultation skills, success will be greater if conscious learning and reflection on performance are employed. Although rarely necessary, it is critical that clinicians who use these approaches believe that patients should have the final say in treatment decisions, and have considered how they would manage a clinically dubious or risky decision in practice. If not, there is a risk that the process of accessing beliefs and relationship building will simply become a sophisticated form of manipulation, and the *compliance* paradigm will live on.

Implication for learning

For educators, this book adds some materials and skills that can be incorporated into an existing patient-centered curriculum, but the importance of exploring learners' values cannot be over-emphasized. Although many learners are happy to learn about patients' thoughts and concerns, and see a value in incorporating these into the care process, some struggle with the notion of giving patients much influence, let alone control, over the treatment decision. We support Stewart and her colleagues' suggestion that patients should be included in the learning process, as they may challenge students' views in a way that no tutor can. There are many excellent existing tried and tested models for analysing and teaching the clinical interview, so what – you may ask – can this approach add to patient-centered medicine, Calgary–Cambridge, SEGUE, Pendleton, Neighbour and others (Pendleton *et al.*, 1984; Neighbour, 1987; Kurtz *et al.*, 1998; Makoul, 2001; Stewart *et al.*, 2003)? Our belief is that we have expanded upon the critical and somewhat elusive component of finding common ground or shared decision making specifically with regard to medication – also known as *concordance*. By linking an understanding of the context (Kleinman's three sectors) with applicable health behavior models (particularly Leventhal's self-regulatory model) and research into clinical interactions and medication use, we have been able to develop and refine a new approach that fits within the larger patient-centered stable. In contrast to the more structured application of shared decision making, we are advocating a process of partnership building in which the clinician's awareness of the patient's perspective is combined with an understanding of the process (including a cognitive and emotional 'testing' phase) and their own knowledge base to enable patients to arrive at the optimal pattern of medication use for them. As with other health-related behavior changes, it is helpful to recognize that adjusting to long-term treatment use is more often a process rather than a discrete decision.

Implication for research

For researchers there are immense challenges ahead. The very notion that we should tell patients what to do has changed, and therefore the way in which interventions are assessed must also be adjusted. Studies or training programs designed to encourage patient-centered prescribing decisions must be judged against individual patients' goals for treatment. These 'complex' interventions will indeed be complex to assess, and some very large-scale studies will be required to throw light on this. However, there are a number of discrete areas about which we need to know more before focussing on evaluation studies.

Relationships

The focus appears to be shifting from task-based approaches (e.g. shared decision making) to one of process. The nature of the clinical relationship and sense of partnership and trust needs to be defined in greater detail conceptually, and ideally measures need to be developed to assess its impact. How is the relationship used and when is this effective or ineffective? How does this play into the cognitive and emotional assessment process for patients?

Attitudes

There is a balance to be struck between patient preference and evidence-based clinical practice in which both patient and clinician have a legitimate interest. However, we know very little about attitudes towards this, their influence on the interaction, or how these attitudes are formed. For instance, how does the perception of legal precedence influence parties' sense of rights and responsibilities and either curb or promote patient involvement? This has implications for the way in which practitioners should be organized and the incentives that are employed. Clinicians without sufficient time will be unable to have the discussions that are necessary to involve patients in decisions. Those who are obliged to operate according to rigid clinical guidelines will not feel able to do so even if they wish to.

'Testing'

If it is accepted that patients do both assess their treatments and act upon those judgements, we need to understand that process in greater detail. It seems feasible to suggest that the cognitive side of this process can be informed through a decision-sharing process, but what if this is not the primary mechanism? Everyone must be familiar with the sense that life is simply too short (perhaps literally) for some decisions to be considered in depth, and consequently choices are made that are based heavily on trust in an individual. How does this emotive element play into the process in different circumstances? How do relationships and other factors influence the type of decision process that is used, and how does this impact upon the testing process? For instance, in what ways does the assessment of low-dose aspirin (a preventive treatment that is usually without side-effects or an obvious effect) compare with a symptomatic treatment such as treatment for asthma?

Skills

Deeper insights into this component of the consultation process are still required, including how and why this can influence decisions and behaviors. Although it has been shown that clinicians can learn new ways of consulting, including these specific techniques, we have no idea how refined these skills need to be in order to be sufficient (Gask et al., 1998; Fallowfield et al., 2002; Edwards et al., 2003c; Dowell et al., 2004). How informed is 'informed'?

Outcomes

It is no longer sufficient to assume that better clinical outcomes, let alone compliance, are the optimal result. We need to assess patients' preferences for their role in the process, as well as their treatment preferences and their priorities for particular outcomes. If an effective attempt to prescribe in a patient-centered manner facilitates an informed choice that a patient feels content with, but produces a poor clinical outcome, this should be recognized as a patient-centered success, not a clinical failure. In order to achieve this, tools such as the Patient-Generated Index will have to be included alongside the more traditional measures of clinical outcomes (Ruta *et al.*, 1994).

Finally, it might be useful to briefly consider what methodologies might be most helpful. There are clearly a number of areas where exploratory qualitative work is required to build theory and map out the pertinent dimensions of components – for instance, the interplay between cognitive and emotive aspects of the decision process. However, this will not be sufficient. It is essential to measure the broad impact of interventions in order to estimate their value and cost-effectiveness. To do so, it will be necessary to overcome a number of challenges in terms of developing new measurement tools and running complex trials with intricate outcome assessments. One attractive solution might be to use trials of simulated practice as a form of pilot to allow explicit experimentation with specific ingredients before very costly intervention trials are attempted. In addition, because so much research has already been conducted in this area, it might be possible to learn more from systematic reviews that integrate the insights gained from qualitative studies with existing data from controlled interventions. However, these approaches are still in their infancy (Thomas *et al.*, 2004).

What next?

This book has been written to encourage clinicians to view medication use as a challenge rather than as a problem that is beyond their influence. Patient participation is increasing, and this will be an enjoyable process if clinicians can embrace it rather than resist it. Patient-centered medicine offers a bridge which can make this possible. From whatever perspective this is viewed, the consultation remains one cornerstone of the therapeutic process, and attempts to research and refine what happens during these critical encounters should be welcomed. We trust that you will enjoy experimenting with some of the ideas and approaches that have been described, and thereby improve your relationships with some patients and, hopefully, their treatment use as well.

References

Abraham C and Sheeran P (2000) Understanding and changing health behaviour: from health beliefs to self-regulation. In: P Norman, C Abraham and M Conner (eds) *Understanding and Changing Health Behaviour: from health beliefs to self-regulation.* Harwood, Singapore.

Adams S, Pill R and Jones A (1997) Medication, chronic illness and identity: the perspective of people with asthma. *Soc Sci Med.* **45:** 189–201.

Ajzen I (1985) From intentions to actions: a theory of planned behaviour. In: J Kuhl and J Beckmann (eds) *Action Control: from cognition to behavior.* Springer, New York.

Ajzen I (1991) The theory of planned behaviour. *Organiz Behav Hum Decision Processes.* **50:** 179–211.

Ajzen I and Fishbein M (1977) Attitude–behaviour relations: a theoretical analysis and review of empirical research. *Psychol Bull.* **84:** 888–918.

Alaszewski A and Horlick-Jones T (2003) How can doctors communicate information about risk more effectively? *BMJ.* **327:** 728–31.

Ambady N, LaPlante D, Nguyen T *et al.* (2002) Surgeons' tone of voice: a clue to malpractice history. *Surgery.* **132:** 5–9.

Anastasio GD, Little JM Jr, Robinson MD *et al.* (1994) Impact of and side-effects on the clinical outcome of patients treated with oral erythromycin. *Pharmacotherapy.* **14:** 229–34.

Armstrong L (2001) *It's Not About the Bike: my journey back to life.* Yellow Jersey Press, London.

Association of the British Pharmaceutical Industry; www.abpi.org.uk/statistics/section.asp?sect=1 (accessed 26 November 2005).

Avis M, Bond M and Arthur A (1997) Questioning patient satisfaction: an empirical investigation in two outpatient clinics. *Soc Sci Med.* **44:** 85–92.

Bain DJG (1977) Patient knowledge and the content of the consultation in general practice. *Med Educ.* **11:** 347–50.

Bajcar J (2006) Task analysis of patients' medication-taking practice and the role of making sense: a grounded theory study. *Res Soc Admin Pharmacy.* **2:** 59–82.

Balint M (1964) *The Doctor, his Patient and the Illness* (2e). Pitman, London.

Banks MH, Beresford SAA, Morrell DC *et al.* (1975) Factors influencing demand for primary medical care in women aged 20–44 years: a preliminary report. *Int J Epidemiol.* **4:** 189–95.

Barber N, Parsons J, Clifford S *et al.* (2004) Patients' problems with new medication for chronic conditions. *Qual Safety Health Care.* **13:** 172–5.

Barry C, Bradley CP, Britten N *et al.* (2000) Patients' unvoiced agendas in general practice consultations: qualitative study. *BMJ.* **320:** 1246–50.

Beardon PHG, McGilchrist MM, McKendrick AD *et al.* (1993) Primary non-compliance with prescribed medication in primary care. *BMJ.* **307:** 846–8.

Beate J, Skorpen J and Malterud K (1997) What did the doctor say – what did the patient hear? Operational knowledge in clinical communication. *Fam Pract.* **14:** 382–6.

Becker LA, Glanz K, Sobel E *et al.* (1986) A randomized trial of special packaging of antihypertensive medications. *J Fam Pract.* **22:** 357–61.

Becker MH, Maiman LA, Kirscht JP *et al.* (1977) Predictions of dietary compliance: a field experiment. *J Health Soc Behav.* **18:** 348–66.

Begg D (1984) Do patients cash prescriptions? An audit in one practice. *J R Coll Gen Pract.* **34:** 272–4.

Benson J and Britten N (2002) Patients' decisions about whether or not to take antihypertensive drugs: qualitative study. *BMJ.* **325:** 873–8.

Bishop G and Converse S (1986) Illness representations: a prototype approach. *Health Psychol.* **5:** 95–114.

Blaxter M (1983) The cause of disease: women talking. *Soc Sci Med.* **17:** 59–69.

Blaxter M (1990) *Health and Lifestyles.* Tavistock/Routledge, London.

Blaxter M and Paterson E (1982) *Mothers and Daughters: a three-generational study of health attitudes and behaviour.* Heinemann, London.

Blenkinsopp A, Bond C, Britten N *et al.* (1997) *From Compliance to Concordance: achieving shared goals in medicine taking.* Merck Sharp and Dohme, Royal Pharmaceutical Society of Great Britain, London.

Bond GG, Aiken LS and Somerville SC (1992) The health belief model and adolescents with insulin-dependent diabetes mellitus. *Health Psychol.* **11:** 190–8.

Boon H, Brown J, Gavin A *et al.* (1999) Breast cancer survivors' perceptions of complementary/alternative medicine (CAM): making the decision to use or not to use. *Qual Health Res.* **9:** 639–53.

Boon H, Stewart M, Kennard MA *et al.* (2000) Use of complementary/alternative medicine by breast cancer survivors in Ontario: prevalence and perceptions. *J Clin Oncol.* **18:** 2515–21.

Boon H, Brown J, Gavin A *et al.* (2003) Men with prostate cancer: making decisions about complementary/alternative medicine. *Med Decis Making.* **23:** 471–9.

Bosley CM, Parry DT and Cochrane GM (1994) Patient with inhaled medication: does combining beta-agonists with corticosteroids improve compliance? *Eur Respir J.* **7:** 504–9.

Brehm S (1981) Freedoms and threats to freedoms. In: S Brehm (ed.) *Psychological Reactance: a theory of freedom and control.* Academic Press, New York.

Bridson J, Hammond C, Leach A *et al.* (2003) Making consent patient centred. *BMJ.* **327:** 1159–61.

British Market Research Bureau (1997) *Everyday Health Care: a consumer study of self-medication in Great Britain.* British Market Research Bureau, London.

Britten N (1994) Patients' ideas about medicines: a qualitative study in a general practice population. *Br J Gen Pract.* **44:** 465–8.

Britten N, Stevenson FA, Barry CA *et al.* (2000) Misunderstandings in prescribing decisions in general practice: qualitative study. *BMJ.* **320:** 484–8.

Britten N, Ukoumunne O and Boulton M (2002) Patients' attitudes to medicines and expectations for prescriptions. *Health Expectations.* **5:** 256–69.

Britten N, Stevenson F and Gafaranga J (2004) The expression of aversion to medicines in general practice consultations. *Soc Sci Med.* **59:** 1495–503.

Brown C and Segal R (1997) The effects of health and treatment perceptions on the use of prescribed medication and home remedies among African American and White American hypertensives. *Soc Sci Med.* **43:** 903–17.

Brown JB, Weston WW and Stewart MA (1989) Patient-centered interviewing. Part 2: finding common ground. *Can Fam Physician.* **35:** 153–7.

Budd R, Hughes I and Smith J (1996) Health beliefs and compliance with antipsychotic medication. *Br J Clin Psychol.* **35:** 393–7.

Butler C, Pill R and Stott N (1998) Qualitative study of patients' perceptions of doctors' advice to quit smoking: implications for opportunistic health promotion. *BMJ.* **316:** 1878–81.

Byrne P and Long B (1989) *Doctors Talking to Patients.* Royal College of General Practitioners, London.

Cabana MD, Powe NR, Wu AW *et al.* (1999) Why don't physicians follow clinical practice guidelines? *JAMA.* **282:** 1458–65.

Calnan M (1989) Control over health and patterns of health-related behaviour. *Soc Sci Med.* **29:** 131–6.

Campion P, Foulkes J, Neighbour R *et al.* (2002) Patient centeredness in the MRCGP video examination: analysis of large cohort. *BMJ.* **325:** 691–2.

Carter S, Taylor D and Levinson R (2003) *A Question of Choice: compliance in medicine taking* (2e). Medicines Partnership, London.

Chewning B and Sleath B (1996) Medication decision-making and management: a client-centered model. *Soc Sci Med.* **42:** 389–98.

Clark NM (2003) Management of chronic disease by patients. *Annu Rev Public Health.* **24:** 289–313.

Colcher IS and Bass JW (1972) Penicillin treatment of streptococcal pharyngitis. *JAMA.* **222:** 657–9.

Conner M and Sparks P (1996) The theory of planned behaviour and health behaviours. In: M Conner and P Noran (eds) *Predicting Health Behaviour: research and practice with social cognition models.* Open University Press, Buckingham.

Cooperstock R and Lennard HL (1979) Some social meanings of tranquilizer use. *Sociol Health Illness.* **1:** 331–47.

Coronary Drug Project Research Group (1980) Influence of adherence to treatment and response of cholesterol on mortality in the Coronary Drug Project. *NEJM.* **303:** 1038–41.

Coulter A (1999) Paternalism or partnership? *BMJ.* **319:** 719–20.

Coulter A (2003) Killing the goose that laid the golden egg? *BMJ.* **326:** 1280–1.

Coulter A, Entwistle VA and Gilbert D (1999) Sharing decisions with patients: is the information good enough? *BMJ.* **318:** 318–22.

Cox K, Stevenson F, Britten NY *et al.* (2004) *A Systematic Review of Communication Between Patients and Health Care Professionals About Medicine-Taking and Prescribing.* GKT Concordance Unit, Guy's King's and St Thomas' School of Medicine, King's College, London.

Coyle J (1997) *Exploring the Meaning of Dissatisfaction with Health Care: towards a grounded theory.* South Bank University, London

Coyle J (1999) Exploring the meaning of 'dissatisfaction' with health care: the importance of 'personal identity threat.' *Sociol Health Illness.* **21:** 95–123.

Coyne T, Olson M, Bradham K *et al.* (1995) Dietary satisfaction correlated with adherence in the Modification of Diet in Renal Disease Study. *J Am Diet Assoc.* **95:** 1301–6.

Cramer JC (1989) How often is medication taken as prescribed? *JAMA.* **261:** 3273–7.

Cromarty J (1996) What do patients think about their consultations? A qualitative study. *Br J Gen Pract.* **46:** 525–8.

Davis DA and Thomson MA (1995) Changing physician performance. A systematic review of the effect of continuing medical education strategies. *JAMA.* **274:** 700–5.

Devereaux PJ, Anderson DR, Gardner MJ *et al.* (2002) Differences between perspective of physicians and patients on anticoagulation in patients with atrial fibrillation: observational study. *BMJ.* **323:** 1–6.

DiMatteo MR, Sherbourne CD, Hays RD *et al.* (1993) Physicians' characteristics influence patients' adherence to medical treatment. Results from the Medical Outcomes Study. *Health Psychol.* **12:** 93–102.

Donovan JL and Blake DR (1992) Patient non-compliance: deviance or reasoned decision-making? *Soc Sci Med.* **34:** 507–13.

Dowell JS and Hudson H (1997) A qualitative study of medication-taking behaviour in primary care. *Fam Pract.* **14:** 369–75.

Dowell JS, Snadden D and Dunbar J (1996) Rapid prescribing change: how do patients respond? *Soc Sci Med.* **43:** 1543–9.

Dowell J, Jones A and Snadden D (2002) Exploring medication use to seek concordance with 'non-adherent' patients: a qualitative study. *Br J Gen Pract.* **52:** 24–32.

Dowell J, Pagliari C and McAleer S (2004) Development and evaluation of a concordance training course for medical practitioners. *Med Teacher.* **26:** 384–6.

Dunnel K and Cartwright A (1972) *Medicine Takers, Prescribers and Hoarders.* Routledge and Kegan Paul, London.

Ebrahim S (1998) Detection, adherence and control of hypertension for the prevention of stroke: a systematic review. *Health Technol Assess.* **2:** 1–78.

Edwards A and Elwyn G (2002) *Evidence-Based Patient Choice: inevitable or impossible?* Oxford University Press, Oxford.

Edwards A, Unigwe S, Elwyn G *et al.* (2003a) Effects of communicating individual risks in screening programmes: Cochrane systematic review. *BMJ.* **327:** 703–7.

Edwards A, Elwyn G, Hood K *et al.* (2003b) The development of COMRADE – a patient-based outcome measure to evaluate the effectiveness of risk communication and treatment decision-making in consultations. *Patient Educ Couns.* **50:** 311–22.

Edwards A, Evans R and Elwyn G (2003c) Manufactured but not imported: new directions for research in shared decision-making support and skills. *Patient Educ Couns.* **50:** 33–8.

Eisenberg L (1977) Distinction between professional and popular ideas of sickness. *Cult Med Psychiatry.* **1:** 9–23.

Elwyn G, Edwards A and Kinnersley P (1999a) Shared decision-making in primary care: the neglected second half of the consultation. *Br J Gen Pract.* **49:** 477–82.

Elwyn G, Gwyn R, Edwards A *et al.* (1999b) Is 'shared decision-making' feasible in consultations for upper respiratory tract infections? Assessing the influence of antibiotic expectations using discourse analysis. *Health Expect.* **2:** 105–17.

Elwyn G, Edwards A, Kinnersley P *et al.* (2000) Shared decision-making and the concept of equipoise: the competencies of involving patients in health care choices. *Br J Gen Pract.* **50:** 892–7.

Elwyn G, Edwards A, Wensing M *et al.* (2001) Shared decision-making observed in clinical practice: visual displays of communication sequence and patterns. *J Eval Clin Pract.* **7:** 211–21.

Elwyn G, Edwards A, Wensing M *et al.* (2003) Shared decision-making: developing the OPTION scale for measuring patient involvement. *Qual Saf Health Care.* **12:** 93–9.

Engel GL (1977) The need for a new medical model: a challenge for biomedicine. *Science.* **196:** 129–36.

Engel GL (1980) The clinical application of the biopsychosocial model. *Am J Psychiatry.* **137:** 535–44.

Fallowfield L, Jenkins V, Farewell V *et al.* (2002) Efficacy of a Cancer Research UK communication skills training model for oncologists: a randomised controlled trial. *Lancet.* **359:** 650–6.

Fallsberg M (1991) *Reflections on Medicines and Medication: a qualitative analysis among people on long-term drugs regimens.* Linkoping University, Sweden.

Finn P and Alcorn J (1986) Noncompliance to hemodialysis dietary regimens: literature review and treatment recommendations. *Rehab Psychol.* **31:** 67–78.

Fishbein M and Ajzen I (1975) *Belief, Attitude, Intention, Behaviour.* Wiley, New York.

Fisher R, Ury W and Patton B (1992) *Getting to Yes* (2e). Random Century, London.

Fletcher SW, Pappius EM and Harper SJ (1979) Measurement of medication in a clinical setting: comparison of three methods in patients prescribed digoxin. *Arch Intern Med.* **139:** 635–8.

Fox W (1983a) Compliance of patients and physicians: experience and lessons from tuberculosis-I. *BMJ.* **287:** 33–5.

Fox W (1983b) Compliance of patients and physicians: experience and lessons from tuberculosis-II. *BMJ.* **287:** 101–5.

Frank A (1995) *The Wounded Storyteller: body, illness and ethics.* University of Chicago Press, Chicago.

Frank A (2001) Can we research suffering? *Qual Health Res.* **11:** 353–62.

Franks PJ, Sian M, Kenchington GF *et al.* (1992) Aspirin usage and its influence on femoro-popliteal vein graft patency. The Femoro-popliteal Bypass Trial Participants. *Eur J Vasc Surg.* **6:** 185–8.

Freeman GK, Horder JP, Howie JGR *et al.* (2002) Evolving general practice consultation in Britain: issues of length and context. *BMJ.* **324:** 880–2.

Gask L, Usherwood T, Thompson H *et al.* (1998) Evaluation of a training package in the assessment and management of depression in primary care. *Med Educ.* **32:** 190–8.

General Medical Council (2002) *Seeking Patients' Consent: the ethical considerations.* General Medical Council, London.

Georgiou A and Bradley C (1992) The development of a smoking-specific locus of control scale. *Psychol Health.* **6:** 227–40.

Gerteis M, Edgman-Levitan S, Daley J et al. (1993) *Through the Patient's Eyes: understanding and promoting patient-centered care*. Jossey-Bass, San Francisco, CA.

Gigerenzer G (2002) *Reckoning with Risk. Learning to live with uncertainty*. Penguin, Harmondsworth.

Gigerenzer G and Edwards A (2003) Simple tools for understanding risks: from innumeracy to insight. *BMJ*. **327**: 741–4.

Gittel JH (2003) *The Southwest Airlines Way*. McGraw-Hill, New York.

Giuffrida A and Torgerson DJ (1997) Should we pay the patient? Review of financial incentives to enhance patient compliance. *BMJ*. **315**: 703–7.

Glynn RJ, Buring JE, Manson JE et al. (1994) Adherence to aspirin in the prevention of myocardial infarction. The Physicians' Health Study. *Arch Intern Med*. **154**: 2649–57.

Godolphin W (2003) The role of risk communication in shared decision making. *Br Med J*. **327**: 692–3.

Gollwitzer PM (1993a) Goal achievement: the role of intentions. *Eur Rev Soc Psychol*. **4**: 141–85.

Gollwitzer PM (1993b) Planning and coordinating action. In: PM Gollwitzer and JA Bargh (eds) *The Psychology of Action*. Guilford Press, New York.

Gore J and Ogden J (1998) Developing, validating and consolidating the doctor–patient relationship: the patient's views of a dynamic process. *Br J Gen Pract*. **48**: 1391–4.

Greenberg RN (1984) Overview of patient with medication dosing: a literature review. *Clin Ther*. **6**: 592–9.

Greene A (2001) Cross-cultural differences in the management of children and adolescents. *Horm Res*. **57**: 75–7.

Greenhalgh T and Hurwitz B (1988) *Narrative-Based Medicine*. BMJ Books, London.

Grilli R and Lomas J (1994) Evaluating the message: the relationship between compliance rate and the subject of a practice guideline. *Med Care*. **32**: 202–13.

Grimshaw J and Russell IT (1993) Do explicit guidelines change medical practice? A systematic review of rigorous evaluations. *Lancet*. **342**: 1317–22.

Gwyn R and Elwyn G (1999) When is a shared decision not (quite) a shared decision? Negotiating preferences in a general practice encounter. *Soc Sci Med*. **49**: 437–47.

Hahn RA and Kleinman A (1983) Belief as pathogen, belief as medicine: 'Voodoo death' and the 'placebo phenomenon' in anthropological perspective. *Med Anthropol Q*. **14**: 16–19.

Harrison JA, Mullen PD and Green LW (1992) A meta-analysis of the health belief model with adults. *Health Educ Res*. **7**: 107–16.

Hassell K, Rogers A, Noyce P et al. (1998) *The Public's Use of Community Pharmacists as a Primary Health Care Resource. The Community Pharmacy Research Consortium Study Report*. The School of Pharmacy and Pharmaceutical Sciences and the National Primary Care Research and Development Centre, University of Manchester, Manchester.

Hawe P and Higgins S (1990) Can medication education improve the drug compliance of the elderly? Evaluation of an in hospital program. *Patient Educ Couns*. **16**: 151–60.

Haynes RB, Sackett DL, Taylor W et al. (1977) Manipulation of the therapeutic regimen to improve compliance: conceptions and misconceptions. *Clin Pharmacol Ther*. **22**: 125–30.

Haynes RB, McKibbon KA and Kanani R (1996) Systematic review of randomised trials of interventions to assist patients to follow prescriptions for medications. *Lancet*. **348**: 383–6.

Hays RD, Kravitz RL, Mazel RM et al. (1994) The impact of patient adherence on health outcomes for patients with chronic disease in the Medical Outcomes Study. *J Behav Med*. **17**: 347–60.

Helman CG (1998) *Culture, Health and Illness*. Butterworth-Heinemann, Oxford.

Henderson JW and Donatelle RJ (2003) The relationship between cancer locus of control and complementary and alternative medicine use by women diagnosed with breast cancer. *Psychooncology*. **12**: 59–67.

Horne R (1997) Representations of medication and treatment: advances in theory and measurement. In: J Weinman and K Petrie (eds) *Perception of Health and Illness*. Harwood Academic, London.

Horne R and Weinman J (1999) Patients' beliefs about prescribed medicines and their role in adherence to treatment in chronic illness. *J Psychosom Res.* **47**: 555–67.

Horne R and Weinman J (2000) Illness cognitions: implications for the treatment of renal disease. In: HM McGee and C Bradley (eds) *Quality of Life Following Renal Failure*. Harwood Academic Publishers, London.

Horne R, Clatworthy J, Polmear A *et al.* (2001) Do hypertensive patients' beliefs about their illness and treatment influence medication adherence and quality of life? *J Hum Hypertens.* **15 (Suppl. 1)**: S65–8.

Horwitz RI and Horwitz SM (1993) Adherence to treatment and health outcomes. *Arch Intern Med.* **153**: 1863–8.

Hoskins G, Neville RG, Smith CR *et al.* (1999) The link between practice nurse training and asthma outcomes. *Br J Commun Nurs.* **4**: 222–8.

Hounsa AM, Godin G, Alihonou E *et al.* (1993) An application of Ajzen's theory of planned behaviour to predict mothers' intention to use oral rehydration therapy in a rural area of Benin. *Soc Sci Med.* **37**: 253–61.

Howie J, Heaney D and Maxwell M (1997) *Measuring Quality in General Practice*. London: Royal College of General Practitioners. Occasional Paper. **75**: 3–7.

Hugh Baron J (2004) Expelling patients 1778. *BMJ.* **328**: 342.

Hughes I, Hill B and Budd R (1997) Compliance with antipsychotic medication: from theory to practice. *J Ment Health.* **6**: 473–89.

Hunter MS, O'Dea I and Britten N (1997) Decision-making and hormone replacement therapy: a qualitative analysis. *Soc Sci Med.* **45**: 1541–8.

Jay S, DuRant RH, Litt IF *et al.* (1984) Riboflavin, self-report and serum norethindrone. Comparison of their use as indicators of adolescent compliance with oral contraceptives. *Am J Dis Child.* **138**: 70–3.

Jones I and Britten N (1998) Why do some patients not cash their prescriptions? *Br J Gen Pract.* **48**: 903–5.

Kaplan S, Greenfield S and Ware J (1989) Assessing the effects of physician–patient interactions on the outcomes of chronic disease. *Med Care.* **27**: 110–27.

Karner A, Goransson A and Bergdahl B (2002) Conceptions on treatment and lifestyle in patients with coronary heart disease – a phenomenographic analysis. *Patient Educ Couns.* **47**: 137–43.

Kleinman A (1980) *Patients and Healers in the Context of Culture*. University of California Press, Berkeley, CA.

Kleinman A (1988) *The Illness Narratives*. Basic Books, New York.

Kleinman A, Eisenberg L and Good B (1978) Culture, illness and care. *Ann Intern Med.* **88**: 251–8.

Kurtz SM, Silverman J and Draper J (1998) *Teaching and Learning Communication Skills in Medicine*. Radcliffe Medical Press, Oxford.

Laederach-Hofmann K and Bunzel B (2000) Non-compliance in organ transplant recipients: a literature review. *Gen Hosp Psychiatry.* **22**: 412–24.

Lahdensuo A (1999) Guided self-management of asthma – how to do it. *BMJ.* **319**: 759–60.

Lassen LC (1991) Connections between the quality of consultations and patient compliance in general practice. *Fam Pract.* **8**: 154–60.

Lau R and Hartman K (1983) Common-sense representations of common illness. *Health Psychol.* **2**: 167–85.

Leventhal H and Nerenz D (1985) The assessment of illness cognition. In: P Karoly (ed.) *Measurement Strategies in Health Psychology*. John Wiley, New York.

Leventhal H, Meyer D and Nerenz D (1980) The common-sense representation of illness danger. In: Rachman S (ed.) *Medical Psychology. Volume 2*. Pergamon, New York.

Leventhal H, Diefenbach M and Lenenthal E (1992) Illness cognition: using common sense to understand treatment adherence and affect cognition interactions. *Cogn Ther Res.* **16:** 143–63.

Ley P (1982) Satisfaction, compliance and communication. *Br J Clin Psychol.* **21:** 241–54.

Ley P (1983) Patients' understanding and recall in clinical communication failure. In: P Ley (ed.) *Doctor–Patient Communication.* London: Academic Press.

Ley P (1988) The problem of patients' non-compliance. In: D Pendleton and J Hasler (eds) *Communicating with Patients: improving communication, satisfaction and compliance* (2e). Chapman and Hall, London.

Lilleyman JS and Lennard L (1996) Non-compliance with oral chemotherapy in childhood leukaemia. *BMJ.* **313:** 1219–20.

Little P, Barnett J, Barnsley L *et al.* (2002) Comparison of acceptability of and preferences for different methods of measuring blood pressure in primary care. *BMJ.* **325:** 258–9.

Logan AG, Milne BJ, Achber C *et al.* (1979) Work-site treatment of hypertension by specially trained nurses. A controlled trial. *Lancet.* **2:** 1175–8.

Lundberg L, Johannesson M, Isacson DGL *et al.* (1998) Effects of user charges on the use of prescription medicines in different socio-economic groups. *Health Policy.* **44:** 123–34.

Macfarlane J, Holmes W, Macfarlane R *et al.* (1997) Influence of patients' expectations on antibiotic management of acute lower respiratory tract illness in general practice: questionnaire study. *Br Med J.* **315:**1211–15.

McDermott I and Jago W (2001) *Brief Neurolinguistic Programming Therapy.* Sage, London.

McDermott MM, Schmitt B and Wallner E (1997) Impact of medication nonadherence on coronary heart disease outcomes. A critical review. *Arch Intern Med.* **157:** 1921–8.

McKenney JM, Munroe WP and Wright JTJ (1992) Impact of an electronic medication aid on long-term blood pressure control. *J Clin Pharmacol.* **32:** 277–83.

McKinstry B and Wang JX (1991) Putting on the style: what patients think of the way their doctor dresses. *Br J Gen Pract.* **41:** 275–8.

McWhinney I (1989) *A Textbook of Family Medicine* (2e). Oxford University Press, Oxford.

Maenpaa H, Javela K, Pikkarainen J *et al.* (1987a) Minimal doses of digoxin: a new marker for compliance to medication. *Eur Heart J.* **8 (Suppl. I):** 31–7.

Maenpaa H, Manninen V and Heinonen OP (1987b) Comparison of the digoxin marker with capsule counting and questionnaire methods for measuring compliance to medication in a clinical trial. *Eur Heart J.* **8 (Suppl. I):** 39–43.

Maher D, Uplekar M, Blanc L *et al.* (2003) Treatment of tuberculosis. *BMJ.* **327:** 822–3.

Makoul G (2001) The SEGUE Framework for teaching and assessing communication skills. *Patient Educ Couns.* **45:** 23–34.

Makoul G, Arnston P and Schofield T (1995) Health promotion in primary care: physician–patient communication and decision-making about prescription medications. *Soc Sci Med.* **41:** 1241–54.

Mant D (1999) Can randomised trials inform clinical decisions about individual patients? *Lancet.* **353:** 743–6.

March L (1994) n of 1 trials comparing a non-steroidal anti-inflammatory drug with paracetamol in osteoporosis. *BMJ.* **309:** 1041–6.

Marinker M (1997) Personal paper: Writing prescriptions is easy. *BMJ.* **314:** 747–8.

Markus H and Wurf E (1997) The dynamic self-concept: a social psychological perspective. *Annu Rev Psychol.* **38:** 299–337.

Matsui D, Hermann C, Klein J *et al.* (1994) Critical comparison of novel and existing methods of assessment during a clinical trial of an oral iron chelator. *J Clin Pharmacol.* **34:** 944–9.

Mead N and Bower P (2002) Patient-centred consultations and outcomes in primary care: a review of the literature. *Patient Educ Couns.* **48:** 51–61.

Meichenbaum D and Turk D (1987) *Facilitating Treatment Adherence.* Plenum, New York.

Mercer SW, Reilly D and Watt GCM (2002) The importance of empathy in the enablement of patients attending the Glasgow Homeopathic Hospital. *BJGP.* **52:** 901–5.

Meredith P and Elliott H (1994) Therapeutic coverage: reducing the risks of partial compliance. *Br J Clin Pract Symp.* **Suppl**. **73**:13–17.

Meyer D, Leventhal H and Gutmann M (1985) Common-sense models of illness: the example of hypertension. *Health Psychol.* **4:** 115–35.

Miller WR and Rollnick S (1991) *Motivational Interviewing* (1e). Guilford, New York.

Montagne M (1988) The metaphorical nature of drugs and drug taking. *Soc Sci Med.* **26:** 417–24.

Montgomery AA and Fahey T (2001) How do patients' treatment preferences compare with those of clinicians? *Qual Health Care.* **10 (Suppl. I):** i39–43.

Montgomery AA, Fahey T and Peters TJ (2003) A factorial randomised controlled trial of decision analysis and an information video plus leaflet for newly diagnosed hypertensive patients. *Br J Gen Pract.* **53:** 446–53.

Moore MA (1988) Improving compliance with antihypertensive therapy. *Am Fam Physician.* **37:** 142–8.

Moos R and Swindle R (1984) The crisis of physical illness: an overview and conceptual approach. In: R Moos (ed.) *Coping with Physical Illness: new perspectives.* Plenum Press, New York.

Morgan M and Watkins C (1988) Managing hypertension: beliefs and responses to medication among cultural groups. *Sociol Health Illness.* **10:** 561–78.

Morisky DE, Levine DM, Green LW *et al.* (1983) Five-year blood pressure control and mortality following health education for hypertensive patients. *Am J Public Health.* **73:** 153–63.

Morris AD, Boyle DIR, McMahon AD *et al.* (1997) Adherence to insulin treatment, glycaemic control, and ketoacidosis in insulin-dependent diabetes mellitus. *Lancet.* **350:** 1505–10.

Morris LS and Schulz RM (1992) Patient compliance – an overview. *J Clin Pharm Ther.* **17:** 283–95.

Morris LS and Schulz RM (1993) Medication: the patient's perspective. *Clin Ther.* **15:** 593–606.

Moynihan R (2004) Drug spending in North America rose by 11% in 2003. *BMJ* **328:** 727.

Neighbour R (1987) *The Inner Consultation. How to develop an effective and intuitive consulting style.* Kluwer, Dordrecht.

Nerenz DR and Leventhal H (1983) Self-regulation theory in chronic illness. In: TG Burish and LA Bradley (eds) *Coping with Chronic Disease.* Academic Press Inc., San Diego, CA.

Ness DEEJ (1994) Denial in the medical interview. *JAMA.* **272:** 1777–81.

Norman P and Bennett P (1998) *Predicting Health Behaviour.* Open University Press, Buckingham.

Norman P, Abraham C and Conner M (2000) *Understanding and Changing Health Behaviour: from health beliefs to self-regulation.* Harwood, Amsterdam.

Novins DK, Beals J, Moore LA *et al.* (2004) Use of biomedical services and traditional healing options among American Indians. *Med Care.* **42:** 670–9.

O'Connor AM, Stacey D, Entwistle V *et al.* (2003a) Decision aids for people facing health treatment or screening decisions. In: *The Cochrane Database of Systematic Reviews. Issue 1.* Update Software, Oxford.

O'Connor A, Legare F and Stacey D (2003b) Risk communication in practice: the contribution of decision aids. *BMJ.* **327:** 736–40.

Ogden J (1996) *Health Psychology: a textbook.* Open University Press, Buckingham.

Ogden J, Ambrose L, Khadra A *et al.* (2002) A questionnaire study of GPs' and patients' beliefs about the different components of patient centeredness. *Patient Educ Couns.* **47:** 223–7.

Paling J (2003) Strategies to help patients understand risks. *Br Med J.* **327:** 745–8.

Paterson C and Britten N (1999) Doctors can't help much: the search for an alternative. *Br J Gen Pract.* **49:** 626–9.

Peabody F (1984) Landmark article 19 March, 1927: The care of the patient. By Francis W Peabody. *JAMA.* **252:** 813–18.

Pearson D and Dudley HAF (1982) Bodily perceptions in surgical patients. *BMJ.* **284:** 1545–6.

Pendleton D, Schofield T, Tate P *et al.* (1984) *The Consultation: an approach to learning and teaching.* Oxford University Press, Oxford.

Pennebaker JW and Watson D (1988) Blood pressure estimation among normotensives and hypertensives. *Health Psychol.* **7:** 309–28.

Perel JM (1988) Compliance during tricyclic antidepressant therapy: pharmacokinetic and analytical issues. *Clin Chem.* **34:** 881–7.

Peterson GM, McLean S and Millingen KS (1984) A randomised trial of strategies to improve patient compliance with anticonvulsant therapy. *Epilepsia.* **25:** 412–17.

Pollock K and Grime J (2000) Strategies for reducing the prescribing of proton pump inhibitors (PPIs): patient self-regulation of treatment may be an under-exploited resource. *Soc Sci Med.* **51:** 1827–39.

Pound P, Britten N, Morgan M *et al.* (2005) Resisting medicines: a synthesis of qualitative studies of medicine taking. *Soc Sci Med.* **61:** 133–55.

Povar GJ, Mantell M and Morris LA (1984) Patients' therapeutic preferences in an ambulatory care setting. *Am J Public Health.* **74:** 1395–7.

Premaratne UN, Sterne JAC, Marks GB *et al.* (1999) Clustered randomised trial of an intervention to improve the management of asthma: Greenwich asthma study. *BMJ.* **318:** 1251–5.

Prochaska JO and DiClemente CC (1983) Stages and processes of self-change of smoking: towards an integrative model of change. *J Consult Clin Psychol.* **51:** 390–5.

Pullar T, Birtwell A, Wiles P *et al.* (1988) Use of a pharmacologic indicator to compare compliance with tablets prescribed to be taken once, twice or three times daily. *Clin Pharmacol Ther.* **44:** 540–5.

Pullar T, Kumar S and Feely M (1989) Compliance in clinical trials. *Ann Rheum Dis.* **48:** 871–5.

Putnam DE, Finney JW, Barkley PL *et al.* (1994) Enhancing commitment improves adherence to a medical regimen. *J Consult Clin Psychol.* **62:** 191–4.

Raynor D (1992) Patient compliance: the pharmacist's role. *Int J Pharm Pract.* **1:** 126–35.

Rehder TL, McCoy LK, Blackwell B *et al.* (1980) Improving medication compliance by counselling and special prescription container. *Am J Hosp Pharm.* **37:** 379–85.

Reibstein J (2002) *Staying Alive: a family memoir.* Bloomsbury, London.

Robertson M (2004) *A discourse analysis of the nature of shared decision-making in general practice consultations.* PhD thesis. University of Dundee, Dundee.

Rollnick S, Kinnersley P and Scott N (1993) Methods of helping patients with behaviour change. *BMJ.* **307:** 188–90.

Rollnick S, Mason P and Butler C (1999) *Health Behavior Change: a guide for practitioners* (8e rev). Churchill Livingstone, Toronto.

Roth HP, Caron HS and Bartholomew P (1996) Measuring intake of a prescribed medication: a bottle count and a tracer technique compared. *Clin Pharmacol Ther.* **11:** 228–36.

Rotter J (1954) *Social Learning and Clinical Psychology.* Prentice-Hall, Englewood Cliffs, NJ.

Rousseau N (2003) Practice-based, longitudinal, qualitative interview study of computerised evidence-based guidelines in primary care. *BMJ.* **326:** 314.

Royal Pharmaceutical Society of Great Britain (1997) *From Compliance to Concordance: towards shared goals in medicine taking.* Royal Pharmaceutical Society of Great Britain, London.

Rubel AJ (1977) *Culture, Disease and Healing: studies in medical anthropology.* Macmillan, New York.

Rubenstein R (1985) *Take It And Leave It: aspects of being ill.* Marion Boyars, New York.

Rudd P, Byyny RL, Zachary V *et al.* (1988) Pill count measures of compliance in a drug trial: variability and suitability. *Am J Hypertens.* **1:** 309–12.

Ruta D, Garrat AM, Leng M *et al.* (1994) A new approach to the measurement of quality of life – the patient-generated index. *Med Care.* **32:** 1109–26.

Sackett D and Haynes RB (1976) *Compliance and Therapeutic Regimens.* Johns Hopkins University Press Ltd, London.

Sackett DL, Haynes RB, Gibson ES *et al.* (1975) Randomised clinical trial of strategies for improving medication compliance in primary hypertension. *Lancet.* **3:** 1205–7.

Sarafino EP (1994) *Health Psychology: biopsychosocial interactions.* John Wiley & Sons, New York.

Satterfield S, Greco PJ, Goldhaber SZ *et al.* (1990) Biochemical markers of compliance in the Physicians' Health Study. *Am J Prev Med.* **6:** 290–4.

Sclar DA and Pharm B (1991) Improving medication compliance: a review of selected issues. *Clin Ther.* **13:** 436–40.

Sclar DA and Skaer TL (1991) Effect of medication utilization review on Medicaid health care expenditures: a case study of patients with non-insulin-dependent diabetes mellitus. *J Res Pharm Economics.* **3:** 75–89.

Sclar DA, Chin A, Skaer TL *et al.* (1991) Effect of health education in promoting prescription refill among patients with hypertension. *Clin Ther.* **13:** 489–95.

Scottish Office (1997) *The National Health Service in Scotland Quarterly Bulletin.* The Stationery Office, Edinburgh.

Shaw C (1999) A framework for the study of coping, illness behaviour and outcomes. *J Adv Nurs.* **29:** 1246–55.

Sheppard B, Hartwick J and Warshaw P (1988) The theory of reasoned action: a meta-analysis of past research with recommendations for modifications and future research. *J Consumer Res.* **15:** 325–43.

SIA Ltd (1995) *Preventing Strokes and Saving Lives.* The Stroke Association, London.

Siegel K and Gorey E (1997) HIV-infected women: barriers to AZT use. *Soc Sci Med.* **45:** 15–22.

Silverman J, Kurtz SM and Draper J (1998) *Skills for Communicating with Patients.* Radcliffe Medical Press, Oxford.

Siminoff LA, Ravdin P, Colabianchi N *et al.* (2000) Doctor–patient communication patterns in breast cancer adjuvant therapy discussions. *Health Expect.* **3:** 26–36.

Skelton J and Pennebaker J (1982) The psychology of physical symptoms and sensations. In: M Jerry and GS Suls (eds) *Social Psychology of Health and Illness.* Lawrence Erlbaum Associates, Hillsdale, NJ.

Skinner TC and Hampson SE (2001) Personal models of diabetes in relation to self-care, well-being and glycemic control. *Diabetes Care.* **24:** 828–33.

Skinner TC, Hampson SE and Fife-Schaw C (2002) Personality, personal model beliefs, and self-care in adolescents and young adults with type 1 diabetes. *Health Psychol.* **21:** 61–70.

Stevenson F, Barry CA, Britten N *et al.* (2000) Doctor–patient communication about drugs: the evidence for shared decision-making. *Soc Sci Med.* **50:** 829–40.

Stevenson F, Britten N, Barry CA *et al.* (2002) Perceptions of legitimacy: the influence on medicine taking and prescribing. *Health.* **6:** 85–104.

Stevenson F, Britten N, Barry CA *et al.* (2003) Self-treatment and its discussion in medical consultations: how is medical pluralism managed in practice? *Soc Sci Med.* **57:** 513–27.

Stewart M (1995) Effective physician–patient communication and health outcomes: a review. *Can Med Assoc J.* **159:** 1423–33.

Stewart M and Roter D (1989) *Communicating with Medical Patients.* Sage Publications, Thousand Oaks, CA.

Stewart M, Brown JB, Weston WW *et al.* (1995) *Patient-Centered Medicine: transforming the clinical method.* Sage Publications, Thousand Oaks, CA.

Stewart M, Brown JB, Weston WW *et al.* (2003) *Patient-Centered Medicine: transforming the clinical method* (2e). Radcliffe Medical Press, Oxford.

Stone AA, Shiffman S, Schwartz JE *et al.* (2002) Patient non-compliance with paper diaries. *BMJ*. **324**: 1193–4.

Stott NCH and Pill RM (1990) 'Advise yes, dictate no': patients' views on health promotion in the consultation. *Fam Pract*. **7**: 125–31.

Strauss A and Corbin J (1990) *Basics of Qualitative Research*. Sage, London.

Strickland BR (1978) Internal–external expectancies and health-related behaviour. *J Consult Clin Psychol*. **46**: 1192–211.

Styron W (2001) *Darkness Visible: a memoir of madness*. Random House, New York.

Sullivan SD, Kreling DH and Hazlet TK (1990) Non-compliance with medication regimens and subsequent hospitalizations: a literature analysis and cost of hospitalization estimate. *J Res Pharm Economics*. **2**: 19–33.

Talbot JS, Webb KA, Hambleton G *et al.* (1998) *Co-operation between health care sectors: developing a novel tool to estimate compliance*. Drug Utilisation Research Group Annual Scientific Meeting, London.

Tashkin DP, Rand C, Nides M *et al.* (1991) A nebulizer chronolog to monitor compliance with inhaler use. *Am J Med*. **91**: 33–6S.

Theunissen NC, de Ridder DT, Bensing JM *et al.* (2003) Manipulation of patient–provider interaction: discussing illness representations or action plans concerning adherence. *Patient Educ Couns*. **51**: 247–58.

Thomas J, Harden A, Oakley A *et al.* (2004) Integrating qualitative research with trials in systematic reviews. *BMJ*. **328**: 1010–12.

Thomas K (2003) Alternative sources of advice: traditional and complementary medicine. In: R Jones, N Britten, L Culpepper *et al.* (eds) *Oxford Textbook of Primary Medical Care*. Oxford University Press, Oxford.

Thomas KB (1987) General practice consultations: is there any point in being positive? *BMJ*. **294**: 1200–2.

Thomas KB (1994) The placebo in general practice. *Lancet*. **344**: 1066–7.

Tobias JS and Souhami RL (1993) Fully informed consent can be needlessly cruel. *BMJ*. **307**: 1199–201.

Towle A and Godolphin W (1999) Framework for teaching and learning informed shared decision-making. *BMJ*. **319**: 766–9.

Townsend A, Hunt K and Wyke S (2003) Managing multiple morbidity in mid-life: a qualitative study of attitudes to drug use. *BMJ*. **327**: 837–40.

Tuckett D, Boulton M, Olson C *et al.* (1985) *Meetings Between Experts*. Tavistock Publications, London.

Urquhart J (2005) Variable compliance and persistence with prescribed drug dosing regimens: implications for benefits, risks, and economics of pharmacotherapy. In: B Strom (ed.) *Pharmacoepidemiology* (4e). John Wiley & Sons, Chichester.

Walker R (1992) Which medication compliance device? *Pharm J*. **249**: 605–7.

Walker R and Wright SE (1985a) Patient compliance and the pharmacist. Part 2. Extent of non-compliance. *Br J Pharm Pract*. **7**: 206–9.

Walker R and Wright SE (1985b) Patient compliance and the pharmacist. *Br J Pharm Pract*. **7**: 166–72.

Watson D and Pennebaker JW (1989) Health complaints, stress and disease: exploring the central role of negative affectivity. *Psychol Rev*. **96**: 234–54.

Weinman J, Petrie K, Moss-Morris R *et al.* (1996) The illness perception questionnaire: a new method for assessing the cognitive representation of illness. *Psychol Health*. **11**: 431–45.

Weston WW and Brown JB (eds) (1995) *Patient-Centered Medicine: transforming the clinical method*. Sage Publications, Thousand Oaks, CA.

Whyte WF (1991) *Participatory Action Research*. Sage, Newbury Park, CA.

Wiles R and Kinmonth A (2001) Patients' understandings of heart attack: implications for prevention of recurrence. *Patient Educ Couns.* **44:** 161–9.

Williams B (1994) Patient satisfaction: a valid concept? *Soc Sci Med.* **38:** 509–16.

Williams B and Grant G (1998) Defining 'people-centredness': making the implicit explicit. *Health Soc Care Community.* **6:** 84–94.

Williams B and Healy D (2001) Perceptions of illness causation among new referrals to a community mental health team: 'explanatory model' or 'exploratory map'? *Soc Sci Med.* **53:** 465–76.

Williams B, Coyle J and Healy D (1998) The meaning of patient satisfaction: an explanation of high reported levels. *Soc Sci Med.* **47:** 1351–9.

Williams R (1983) Concepts of health: an analysis of lay logic. *Sociology.* **17:** 185–205.

Williams S, Weinman J and Dale J (1998) Doctor–patient communication and patient satisfaction: a review. *Fam Pract.* **15:** 480–92.

Wilson P and McNamara J R (1982) How perceptions of a simulated physician–patient interaction influence intended satisfaction and compliance. *Soc Sci Med.* **16:** 1699–708.

Winefield HR, Murrell TG and Clifford J (1995) Process and outcomes in general practice consultations: problems in defining high-quality care. *Soc Sci Med.* **41:** 969–75.

Wong BSM and Norman DC (1987) Evaluation of a novel medication aid, the calendar blister-pak, and its effect on drug compliance in a geriatric outpatient clinic. *J Am Geriatr Soc.* **35:** 21–6.

Young A (1981) When rational men fall sick: an inquiry into some assumptions made by medical anthropologists. *Cult Med Psychiatry.* **5:** 317–35.

Index